Breathing Lessons

Breathing Lessons

A Doctor's Guide to Lung Health

MeiLan K. Han, MD

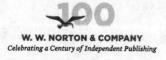

W. W. NORTON & COMPANY
Celebrating a Century of Independent Publishing

Breathing Lessons is intended as a general information resource. It is not a substitute for individual professional medical advice, and no recommendation in the book is intended to substitute for any prescribed medication or course of treatment. Please consult a pulmonologist or primary care provider for evaluation of any symptom that may indicate a lung condition.

The names of all patients mentioned in this book have been changed and potentially identifying details changed or omitted.

Copyright © 2022 by MeiLan K. Han

First published as a Norton paperback 2023

For information about permission to reproduce selections from this book, write to Permissions, W. W. Norton & Company, Inc., 500 Fifth Avenue, New York, NY 10110

For information about special discounts for bulk purchases, please contact
W. W. Norton Special Sales at specialsales@wwnorton.com or 800-233-4830

Manufacturing by LSC Communications, Harrisonburg
Book design by Daniel Lagin
Production manager: Lauren Abbate

Library of Congress Cataloging-in-Publication Data

Names: Han, MeiLan K., author.
Title: Breathing lessons : a doctor's guide to lung health / MeiLan K. Han, M.D.
Description: First edition. | New York, N.Y. : W. W. Norton & Company, [2022] |
    Includes bibliographical references and index.
Identifiers: LCCN 2021022394 | ISBN 9780393866629 (hardcover) |
    ISBN 9780393866636 (epub)
Subjects: LCSH: Lungs—Physiology. | Respiration. | Respiratory organs—Physiology.
Classification: LCC QP121 .H315 2022 | DDC 612.2/4—dc23
LC record available at https://lccn.loc.gov/2021022394

ISBN 978-1-324-06590-6 pbk.

W. W. Norton & Company, Inc., 500 Fifth Avenue, New York, N.Y. 10110
www.wwnorton.com

W. W. Norton & Company Ltd., 15 Carlisle Street, London W1D 3BS

1 2 3 4 5 6 7 8 9 0

For my patients: past, present, and future

Contents

Introduction

I grew up in a small town in Idaho where my father worked as a nuclear engineer and my mother as a nurse and teacher. I attended the University of Washington for medical school, as do many aspiring physicians from the less populous northwestern states. Having grown up and trained in rural areas, I intended to go back to Idaho to serve a small-town community where the need for well-trained doctors is large. But somewhere along the way, I was drawn to pulmonary and critical care medicine, in particular researching how we can better diagnose and treat lung disease. I wanted to contribute to the greater societal good, and in pulmonary medicine I felt that I could have the greatest impact.

I am now a professor of medicine in the Division of Pulmonary and Critical Care at the University of Michigan Medical Center. As a clinician, I have spent the last 20 years taking care of thousands of patients with a huge variety of lung problems.

As a researcher, I have focused on gathering and analyzing data to help the global community better understand who becomes sick, how and why they become sick, and what we can do about it. To this end, I have enrolled patients into clinical trials. I have worked with others at my institution to develop imaging software that helps us better visualize the lungs and quantify the amount of disease. I have also partnered with the National Institutes of Health to explore how we can better set research agendas for the future, and consulted with pharmaceutical companies to help develop new treatments for patients.

Through all of these interactions, what has struck me is both how little most of my patients understand about how the lungs work and how little attention lung disease receives, especially compared with other health conditions. That is, until the youth vaping epidemic and then the COVID-19 pandemic struck. Suddenly, many had questions about how the lungs work, what smoking and vaping do to the lungs, what exactly causes oxygen levels to drop, and how devices like mechanical ventilators support failing lungs.

The lungs are incredible. This single organ provides our bodies with life-giving oxygen, rids us of excess carbon dioxide, and regulates the blood's acid-base balance while also moving air past our vocal cords and nose, allowing us to speak, sing, and even smell. In reading this book, I hope you share my excitement in understanding how your lungs work. But one of the problems that the lungs face is that they actually work a bit too well. By this I mean they can suffer quite a bit of damage before anyone notices. Unfortunately, this also means that lung disease is too often ignored by both patients and physicians until late in the disease course. In this book, I address the challenge human lungs face in being constantly exposed to the environment and the crucial role they play in protecting us. I explore all the things that can go wrong with the lungs. (Spoiler alert: There are many!) And I explain the process lung doctors go through in diagnosing and treating lung conditions.

Perhaps most importantly, I want to help you understand how you can protect your lungs. Beyond telling people "not to smoke," this isn't something we as physicians do enough of. We don't talk about lung health, and that's a problem. We don't give our patients the information they need to preserve their lung capacity, which is crucial to preserving overall health. Lung health begins in the womb and extends throughout childhood and into adulthood, when we finally reach peak lung function. If you are a parent, this is information you need to know to protect your children. If you are a young adult, this is information you need to set yourself up for a lifetime of health. And if you are a patient or have a friend or family member living with lung disease, this book will hopefully help you have more informed conversations with your health care providers.

I also offer my perspective on the peculiar position the field of lung medicine finds itself in and how I believe we got here. Lower respiratory infections, primarily caused by bacterial infections, are the leading cause of death among children worldwide. Chronic obstructive pulmonary disease (COPD) is the third leading cause of death worldwide, and yet it continues to fly under the public's radar. Lung diseases remain poorly recognized and poorly understood. Factors that contribute to lung disease, such as air pollution, should be front and center in the mind of everyone, and yet they are not. Every doctor's office should have a spirometer to measure lung function, and yet they do not. The amount of money invested into lung research should be proportionate to the number of patients living with lung disease, and yet it is not.

The good news is that the tide may be turning. The first step is understanding. I hope that this book helps in that effort and that the information in it helps make your life and the lives of those around you better.

Breathing Lessons

Chapter 1

How the Lungs Work

Breathe in. Breathe out. The act seems simple enough. Try it for a moment. Feel more relaxed? The average person takes over 600 million breaths in their lifetime without giving the activity a second thought. Breathing is an unapplauded marathon. Being able to breathe easily is something most of us take for granted. That is, until it isn't. Nothing is more panic inducing than not being able to breathe. For my entire life, not being able to breathe has been a recurring nightmare. Each time the dream differs in its details, but it always ends the same. I've been trapped by something or someone, and I go to scream. I can't breathe. I can't make even a sound, and I panic. I wake up. And so it is for the millions of individuals living with chronic lung disease, anxiety with every breath.

Yet as important as the lungs are, it is remarkable how poorly understood they are by most people. Most people have at least a rudimentary understanding of how the heart works, but the lungs remain a black box. I have spent nearly 20 years of my life as a pulmonologist, and regardless of the patient's background or level of education, the first visit is always similar. We sit down together, I get out a piece of paper, and I start drawing. I map out the upside-down treelike structure of the lungs. I explain where the air goes and, perhaps most confusingly, how the blood goes from the heart to the lungs to exchange carbon dioxide for oxygen and back to the heart before being pumped out to the rest of the body. While I am a physician and a researcher, I am also an educator. I firmly believe that my patients must understand how their lungs work. It is only then that they can be true partners in recovering from disease and preserving their own lung health.

If you are among those who do not understand how the lungs work, you are in good company. The purpose of breathing remained a mystery for centuries. More than 2,000 years ago, the Greek physician Hippocrates recognized that breathing was a sign of life. But in the absence of anatomic dissection, he taught his students that the soul originated from air (pneuma) that was inspired through the nose into the brain. Around the same time, the philosopher Plato taught that breath entered the body through the skin and exited via the nose. Even after human and animal dissection became common practice, the flow of blood from the heart to the lungs and back to the heart was not sorted out until the 1600s. It wasn't until 1775, when oxygen was discovered by the French chemist Antoine Lavoisier, that it was recognized that the lungs exist to perform two primary functions: to take in oxygen and to expel carbon dioxide. And even today, there is much still to discover.

Lung Structure

The lungs sit in the chest, tucked on top of, around, and behind the heart. If you were to open up the chest cavity and take out the heart, you would realize how perfectly molded the lungs are to their surroundings. They take on the exact shape of the encasement the ribs form around them. The right lung has three lobes (upper, middle, and lower), while the left lung has two lobes (upper and lower) and a cutout, called the *cardiac notch*, where the heart sits. With every breath, the lungs slide back and forth around the heart.

When within the living body, the human lungs weigh roughly 900 to 1,000 grams (about 33 ounces), nearly half of which is blood. On average, the adult human lung can hold up to 6 liters of air when fully inflated, although this varies based on factors such as height and sex. Air enters the lungs through the trachea and then splits into the right and left mainstem bronchi. These bronchi then branch into smaller and smaller air passages called *bronchioles* that ultimately terminate into tiny air-filled sacs called *alveoli*, which are the gas exchange units for the lungs.

The airway branching structure is a beautiful example of a naturally occurring fractal, a shape that repeats at progressively smaller and smaller scales. Fractals demonstrate self-similarity, where each small shape resembles the original larger structure. Nature is full of fractals; a familiar one is the branching pattern of a tree.

For trees, each branch is a copy of the one that came before it. For the lungs, the trachea is the main airway, which can be thought of as the trunk. The trachea then subdivides into smaller and smaller airways, just like the branches on a tree, for 16 divisions. For the next 7 divisions, we begin to see alveolar sacs, the lung's gas exchange units, added to the branches, just like leaves on a tree. For both trees and the lungs, their fractal nature allows them to do one thing really well: maximize the surface area available to exchange gas. Trees pull in carbon dioxide from the air and release oxygen, while humans take in oxygen and eliminate carbon dioxide. Just like tree branches, the airways

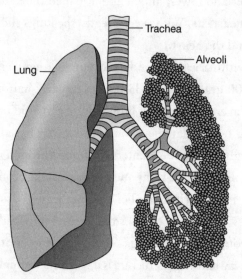

Structure of the human respiratory system, resembling an upside-down tree. The main airway is the trachea, which then splits into a right and left mainstem. The right lung has three lobes, while the left lung has two. The airways further subdivide until they terminate in the tiny gas exchange units of the lungs: the air sacs, or alveoli.

themselves do not participate in gas exchange. Rather, the alveoli function as our "leaves."

Inside the human body, healthy human lungs are a wonder to behold. They glisten a soft pink. With each breath, the twin balloons expand and contract, gently slipping back and forth inside their shell formed by the ribs. Yet unlike balloons, the lungs are not perfectly round. Rather, their elegant shape is a perfect impression of the home in which they live. The top is round while the inner and under surfaces are concave to accommodate the heart and diaphragm. Their lowest point actually comes to a delicate tip like the edge of a bell, and they miraculously retain this fragile shape even when removed from the body.

Unhealthy lungs, however, are frankly grotesque. Diseased, fibrotic lungs shrink and gnarl with scar tissue. In other instances, wart-like bubbles appear on the surface where air has become permanently trapped. Factors such as air pollution or tobacco smoke turn the once pristinely pink tissue to a sickly gray, the surface pockmarked with black deposits. And in lungs destroyed by emphysema, like a parasite feeding on a host, the lung's flesh is eaten from the inside out.

Few, however, have borne witness to the lung's true beauty, as it is not possible to fully appreciate outside its native environment. Once cut, the lung immediately deflates. I remember the first time we took my son to the beach, and we happened upon some unrecognizable blue threads in the sand. My son wanted to know what they were. I explained to him that they were jellyfish, even though they looked nothing like the graceful creatures he had seen in aquariums. It is similar with the lungs.

For those who study lung structure, this deflation makes it difficult to make exact measurements of the lung's microstructures. To overcome this challenge, my research group reinflates lungs with air and then flash-freezes them with liquid nitrogen so that we can study the frozen sections with a highly specialized microscope. While the healthy lung looks like a dense sponge, lungs affected by emphysema look more like a loofah sponge due to destruction of the alveolar air sacs. In fact, for some emphysematous lungs I have studied, the holes are so big and there is so little connective tissue left that the frozen lung crumbles in my hand.

The underlying support structure for the airways consists of cartilage and smooth muscle. Oddly, the biological purpose of airway smooth muscle is unknown. It may help to stiffen the airways against external compression, say during a cough, but what the airway smooth muscle is best known for is its contribution to disease. For patients with conditions that result in airway inflammation like asthma, the smooth muscle constricts. Along with inflammation in the lining of the airway, this constriction makes the resulting air passages narrower. In some patients with more severe asthma, the amount of airway smooth muscle actually increases, further worsening airway narrowing. During exhalation, air pressure in the alveoli temporarily increases, driving the air out toward the opening of the lungs, where air pressure is lower. However, in regions where airways are narrowed, they may close before the air is actually expelled, thereby trapping air in the lung. We call this airflow obstruction.

The smallest airways, the bronchioles, terminate in the lung's gas exchange units, the alveoli. The average adult lung is only about 24 centimeters long in a normal breathing state, about the size of a small loaf of bread. Yet the total surface area of the lung is between 80 and 100 square meters, the size of one side of a tennis court. More than 50 percent of the lung alveoli reside in the outer third of the lung, which is why if you've ever looked at a chest X-ray, the outer edges of the lung appear mostly black. Air appears as black on chest X-rays because there is nothing to stop the X-ray beam from hitting the film (at least before the advent of digital X-rays!). It is only where the soft tissues or bony tissues absorb X-rays that we see the white shadows on the image.

The alveoli have been described as tiny air-filled sacs. Though this description brings to mind a spherical structure, polygonal would be more accurate. Each alveolus shares a wall with the adjacent alveolus. These shared walls help provide the alveolus support. Under a microscope, the cut surface of the lung has an almost honeycomb-like appearance. The alveoli are why the lungs exist. This is where the lungs do the their two most important jobs: to take in oxygen and get rid of carbon dioxide. To stay alive, humans need oxygen. Oxygen is the ignition our cells need to turn food into a usable form of energy. Starve the body of oxygen, and organs such as the brain begin to die within 5 minutes. But our lungs also need to rid the body of carbon dioxide, the waste product of our tiny cellular engines. Too much carbon dioxide can actually render a person unconscious. For some patients with chronic lung diseases such as COPD, admissions to the hospital with carbon dioxide poisoning are not uncommon. We call this hypercapnia. It is ironic that the term *capnia* comes from the Greek word *kapnos*, meaning "smoke." Carbon dioxide is a principal component of tobacco smoke, which is a common cause of COPD.

The alveoli are constructed to maximize gas exchange. To accomplish this feat, their walls are extremely thin, only one cell thick. The primary structural cell of the alveolus, called the *type I pneumocyte*, looks like a very, very flat egg, where the nucleus of the cell is the yolk. The type I cell is only 50 microns wide, about the width of a human hair, but less than 0.2 microns thick. Each alveolus is wrapped in a dense network of tiny blood vessels called capillaries that surround the alveoli. The capillaries are so small that red blood cells must flow through single file. This maximizes the contact between red blood cells and the air present within the alveoli. Within a span of 45 seconds, the lungs are able to process the body's entire volume of blood in this manner, with nearly every red blood cell passing through the tiniest of alveolar capillaries. So anything that fills the alveoli with fluid, like pneumonia, or damages them, as we can see in conditions like pulmonary fibrosis, reduces the lung's ability to take up oxygen.

The alveoli also contain a rarer second cell type, the type II pneumocyte. This cell type makes up only 5 percent of the alveolar surface but performs a crucial function. The type II cell produces a compound called *surfactant* that is part of the fluid lining the alveolar surface. Surfactant is a complex substance made of lipids and proteins. It is the lung's wonder molecule. Surfactant reduces the surface tension in the alveoli. Why is this important? While this is a simplification, think about the alveolus like a bubble. The pressure required for inflation is determined first by the size of the bubble and second by its surface tension. The smaller the bubble, the more pressure is required to inflate it. Think about how hard it is to get the first breath of air into a balloon, compared with how much easier it is once the balloon gets larger. The alveoli are very small, but some are still larger than others. That size difference theoretically means that larger alveoli will open more easily than smaller alveoli, sending air from small alveoli to larger ones, leading to collapse of smaller alveoli and very uneven inflation.

The other factor influencing inflation pressure is surface tension. The surface tension of water is high enough that it rarely allows for bubble formation unless we add a soap to lower that tension. Not only does surfactant lower surface tension like a soap, but this effect is even greater in smaller alveoli than in larger ones. By lowering the surface tension, surfactant reduces the amount of pressure needed to inflate the "alveolar bubbles," particularly the smaller ones. So surfactant helps all alveoli to stay open during both inhalation and exhalation. While multiple factors, such as their shared walls and connective tissue "cables," help to keep alveoli open, scientists generally agree that surfactant plays an important role.[1]

The clearest evidence for the importance of surfactant comes from the birth of premature infants. Fetuses do not begin to produce surfactant until somewhere between 24 and 28 weeks gestation. In 1963, Jacqueline Bouvier Kennedy and President John Fitzgerald Kennedy gave birth to a baby boy, Patrick, at 35 weeks after a placental disruption. Not having enough surfactant poses a significant risk for the lungs of premature babies.

Just two days later, Patrick died of respiratory complications, then called *hyaline membrane disease*, so named for the wax-like membranous layers found coating the lungs of such infants. Although the role of surfactant in reducing surface tension had been discovered in the 1950s, within a year after this tragic event, trials with synthetic surfactants began in earnest. Today we have multiple surfactant medications to treat infants who develop *respiratory distress syndrome*, as it is now called. These treatments have cut neonatal mortality from respiratory distress syndrome by up to 40 percent.[2]

Intertwined among the treelike structure of the lung are blood vessels. In fact, there are *two* completely different sets of blood vessels that supply the lung. The first are the bronchial arteries, the primary blood supply delivering oxygen and nutrients to the trachea and larger airways. These bronchial arteries originate from the biggest artery in the body, the aorta. Most commonly two bronchial arteries arise on the left and one on the right, although significant variation in the takeoff points for these arteries is common. Fascinatingly, however, when patients undergo lung transplants, this blood supply is *not* restored at the time of transplant. It is the *only* transplanted organ whose own arterial blood supply is not reestablished at the time of surgery.

This is only possible because of the lung's second blood supply, the pulmonary arteries and veins. These blood vessels exist in service not primarily to the lungs but rather to the rest of the body. Based on years of conversations with patients, this is probably one of the least understood concepts of lung biology. By definition, arteries deliver blood away from the heart and veins deliver blood to the heart. So the bronchial arteries carry oxygenated blood to the lungs and the bronchial veins return deoxygenated blood to the heart. On the other hand, the pulmonary arteries are unique in that they deliver *deoxygenated* blood from the right chamber of the heart to the lungs, where red blood cells exchange carbon dioxide for oxygen. The pulmonary veins then deliver these newly recharged, *oxygenated* blood cells to the left side of the heart, where they can be pumped out to the rest of the body.

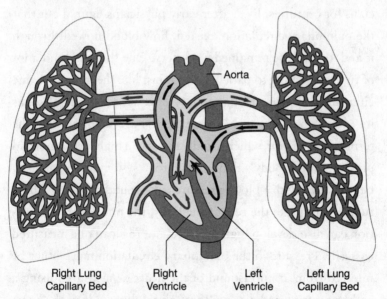

Schematic of pulmonary circulation. Oxygen-depleted blood is returned by the body to the right side of the heart. The heart then pumps that blood to the lungs via the pulmonary arteries. Within the lung's capillary beds, the blood absorbs oxygen and releases carbon dioxide. Oxygen-enriched blood is then returned to the left side of the heart by the pulmonary veins. From the left side of the heart, blood is pumped into the aorta and on to the rest of the body.

So the lungs are the only part of the body where arteries are carrying oxygen-depleted blood and veins are carrying oxygen-enriched blood. One could liken red blood cells to little batteries and the lungs to the battery charger. Inside the lungs, the hemoglobin molecules in the red blood cells drop off carbon dioxide and pick up oxygen. Once the blood is "recharged," it travels back to the heart, where it can once again be sent to deliver oxygen throughout the body.

The pulmonary arteries and veins together are called the pulmonary circulation system. This system has confused physicians for centuries. Even after early physicians figured out that the pulmonary circulation existed, how blood flowed through it and its purpose remained a mystery. One thing I spend a lot of time explaining to patients is that just like the main systemic circulatory system, the pulmonary circulatory system also has its own "blood pressure." Most people are familiar with the term *hypertension*, which usually refers to a higher than normal pressure in the body's main circulatory system and can easily be measured with a blood pressure cuff around the arm. Unfortunately, just like the rest of the body, the pulmonary circulation can also develop high pressure, but this can't be measured as easily. Pressure in the pulmonary circulation must either be inferred from an ultrasound of the heart or measured using a catheter introduced directly through the right side of the heart and into the pulmonary arteries of the lung.

Compared with the left side of the heart, the right side is relatively weak and not built to withstand very high pressures. Normally, the right side of the heart doesn't have to work very hard because the pulmonary circulation is a relatively low pressure system. To provide some context, while a normal blood pressure for the systemic circulation is 120/80 mm Hg, a normal pressure for the pulmonary circulation is closer to 25/10 mm Hg. When disease causes pressure in this circuit to be elevated, this is called *pulmonary hypertension*, which unfortunately is much more difficult to treat than systemic hypertension.

The pulmonary circulation performs several remarkable additional functions. This reservoir of blood in the lung provides a buffer against sudden changes in output from the right side of the heart, so that blood has a place to go temporarily, allowing the left side of the heart to catch up and match output. This vascular bed also serves one of the most important and protective filter functions of the entire body.

I first learned about this critical function of the lung during my anesthesia rotation in medical school. Anyone who has ever spent time in an operating room knows that the anesthesiologists are largely hidden behind a curtain in Wizard of Oz fashion while the surgeons operate in their protected sterile field on the other side of the curtain. Behind the curtain, I came to look forward to my daily real-time anatomy and physiology lessons. During one such case, I was watching a unit of fresh frozen plasma (blood product enriched with clotting factors) filter down through an IV line when I noticed a small amount of clotted material drifting through the tubing toward the patient. I hastily grabbed the IV tubing and pinched it. I naively pointed out that we had an emergency and needed to stop this clot from entering the body. I knew as well as any other medical student that even very small clots that lodge into tiny blood vessels can cause strokes and heart attacks. I will never forget when the attending anesthesiologist grinned at me from behind his operating room mask and exclaimed, "This is what the lungs are for!" And of course, he was right. That little clot would never cause any real harm. The clot would lodge itself into a tiny blood vessel in the pulmonary circulation. Only after the blood vessels become incredibly small do these tributaries rejoin into the larger pulmonary veins that deliver blood back to the left side of the heart and on to the rest of the body. The clot would be caught in these tiny passageways until the body had time to dissolve it.

Clots that are released from the left side of the heart do have potential to cause significant problems, such as strokes. But for patients with normal anatomy, tiny clots leaving the right side of the heart will be filtered by the lungs before they can do any damage. This is not to say, however, that the lungs have infinite capacity for clots. Clots developing in the venous system of the legs are quite common, particularly in patients who have had recent surgery or are immobile. It is not uncommon for these to break loose, enter the right side of the heart, and become trapped in the lung. If these clots are big enough, they can cause damage to the lung. These are called *pulmonary emboli*. If emboli become too numerous or too large, they can cut off blood supply to the lungs, resulting in a pulmonary infarction, akin to a myocardial infarction. They can also cause strain on the right side of the heart and lead to heart failure. Pulmonary emboli are never good, but the body does have this "built-in" protective mechanism that prevents such clots from threatening the blood supply of the brain and other organs.

It is interesting to note that in the upright human, more blood is distributed to the lower lung zones simply due to gravity. Studies done on astronauts show that in outer space, blood flow is much more evenly distributed throughout the lungs.[3] But on earth, where we have gravity, when lying on one's back, more blood is distributed toward the back of the lungs. In everyday life, this is less relevant, but when patients are sick, particularly in the ICU, this concept becomes important. If a person remains lying on their back for a prolonged period of time, the part of the lung in the back tends to become more poorly aerated. We call this atelectasis. The resulting mismatch between alveoli that are poorly ventilated but well supplied with blood can be partially corrected by rolling sick patients onto their stomachs. In the ICU we call this "prone" positioning. This technique can help improve a patient's blood oxygen content by sending more blood to parts of the lung that are better aerated. While this practice has been employed by ICU physicians since the 1970s, it has become more widely known given its recent use in treating patients with COVID-19.

Yet the pulmonary circulation does have some ability to help redirect blood flow. The pulmonary arteries can shift blood flow away from regions of the lung with lower levels of oxygen toward regions of the lung that are better oxygenated. This ability is called *hypoxic vasoconstriction* because the blood vessels constrict in areas of low oxygen. How the blood vessels do this is still somewhat of a mystery, but the fact that the lungs can do it is incredibly important for maximizing oxygenation of the blood, particularly if certain regions of the lung are not performing well. For instance, if a patient has an infection of the lung in one region (pneumonia), then it would be advantageous to redirect blood away from that area. As the alveoli fill with fluid, the oxygen delivered to the capillaries also drops. The blood vessels respond by redirecting blood to better-oxygenated portions of the lung.

Perhaps the most intriguing example of hypoxic vasoconstriction occurs at birth. In the womb, the lungs are bathed in amniotic fluid. Oxygen is instead delivered from the mother's placenta to the fetus via the umbilical cord. Because of this, the entire pulmonary vasculature remains constricted, and much of the fetus's blood bypasses the lungs completely by way of a strictly fetal structure known as the ductus arteriosus. However, when a baby is born and takes in its first breaths, oxygen rushes in and the resistance in the pulmonary vascular circuit precipitously drops. Immediately the pulmonary blood vessels relax and blood surges into the lungs. Through this highly sophisticated mechanism, within a matter of moments babies are transformed from underwater "placental breathers" to "air breathers," allowing newborn infants to survive outside the womb.

The lung is wrapped in a thin membrane called the *visceral pleura*. The thoracic cavity that the lungs sit inside is also wrapped in a thin membrane, the parietal pleura. The space in between the two is called the *pleural space*. Under normal conditions, a very small amount of fluid exists in the pleural space (roughly 6 to 12 milliliters of fluid in a 60-kilogram individual). This configuration allows the lungs to glide along the parietal pleura quite easily as the lungs expand and contract with inspiration and exhalation. As with many of the lung's mysteries, most of us remain unaware these structures even exist until there is a problem. However, certain conditions, like heart failure or pneumonia, can cause fluid to build up outside the lung in the pleural space. If inflammation is present, such as with pneumonia, there may be significant pain. Unlike the rest of the lung, the visceral and parietal pleurae are well innervated with pain fibers. Hence, pain with breathing is sometimes referred to as "pleurisy." The term *pleurisy* is very nonspecific, and the condition can be caused by a wide range of abnormalities. The rest of the lung is not well innervated with pain fibers. So when patients complain to me about pain they think is coming from the lungs, if I cannot find evidence of pleural inflammation, I frequently hunt for other causes of pain, like irritation of the muscles or bones in the chest wall. Because nerve branches from multiple internal organs converge into central nerve roots leading to the brain, sometimes the brain is unable to distinguish where pain is coming from. We call this referred pain.

The other instance where the pleural space makes itself known is when the lung develops a hole, otherwise known as a pneumothorax. Air escapes through the hole and begins to fill the pleural space. As the air outside the lung accumulates, it can cause the lung to collapse. Under the worst possible conditions, the air leak can become so large and the volume of air trapped outside the lung so great that it begins to compress the heart and the opposite lung. This type of situation, known as a tension pneumothorax, can be a real medical emergency requiring immediate decompression. If such a situation is suspected, we can place a needle through the chest wall for immediate decompression, allowing more time to introduce a tube into the chest cavity to provide a release valve for the trapped air. Fortunately, this type of pneumothorax is rare, although pneumothoraces in general are not rare. Sometimes these holes develop due to an underlying lung condition, but sometimes these events just happen. "Spontaneous" pneumothoraces that occur for no apparent reason are more common in men than in women. In fact, it is well recognized among physicians that those at greatest risk for spontaneous pneumothorax have similar characteristics: tall, thin, and often adolescent men. In some cases, no treatment is needed. If the amount of air is large or getting worse, we may insert a tube into the pleural space to drain the air. In rare cases, more significant surgery may be needed to help the lung stay inflated.

The Mechanics of Respiration

How we breathe is not something most of us ever stop to contemplate. Breathing mechanics are also not particularly intuitive. Theoretically, there are two ways air could get into the lungs. Air could either be pushed in (positive-pressure breathing) or pulled in (negative-pressure breathing). In both cases, air flows from an area of high pressure to an area of low pressure. In the former, a high-pressure area is created, forcing air to a lower-pressure area. In the latter, a low-pressure area is created, pulling air from the higher-pressure area. For instance, frogs are positive-pressure breathers. Frogs actively gulp air into their mouths, squeeze their mouths tight, and push air from their mouths into the lungs. Forcing air into the lungs is also how mechanical ventilators work. On the other hand, humans are negative-pressure breathers. Our primary breathing muscle, the diaphragm, sits underneath the lungs. In its rest position, it forms twin domes, one underneath each lung. When we inhale, the domes contract and flatten. The diaphragm pulls the lungs down with it, causing the lungs to expand. Air rushes into the low-pressure cavity created by the expanded lungs. During exhalation, the diaphragm relaxes upward. The pressure inside the lungs becomes slightly positive as compared to atmospheric pressure, and air rushes out.

Take a breath in, and now let it out. Stop at the point where it feels natural to stop. We call the volume of air left in the lung at this exact spot *functional residual capacity (FRC)*. For an average adult, there is about 2.5 liters of air in the lung at FRC. During most of the respiratory cycle, the lungs act like a rubber band pulling inward. The tendency of the lung to collapse inward is called *elastic recoil*. At the same time, the chest wall also has a recoil force directed outward. FRC occurs at the exact point where these two opposing forces are perfectly balanced. Where FRC occurs matters because in diseases like emphysema, in which the lungs lose their elasticity, the balance point at which FRC occurs is greater and the lungs become too big. Unfortunately, this pushes the diaphragm down. When a person with emphysema breathes in, the diaphragm is already so low, it has nowhere to go. They are already flat, making it very difficult for patients to breathe. On the other hand, for patients with diseases that scar the lungs, sometimes called *pulmonary fibrosis*, the forces drawing the lung in become too great and the lung shrinks (lower FRC).

There are other muscles besides the diaphragm that participate in breathing, including the intercostal muscles between the ribs and many of the muscles in the chest, neck, back, and abdomen that create a girdle around the chest cavity. When the lung is diseased, patients must rely more on these accessory muscles to help with the extra burden of breathing. These other muscles also come more into play during forceful inhalations and exhalations. For instance, an even greater exhalation can occur by contracting the accessory respiratory muscles, including the intercostal muscles, to increase pressure in the abdominal cavity, force the diaphragm up, and push additional air out. However, it is impossible for anyone to force all the air from their lungs. Even at maximum exhalation, the average adult has about 1.2 liters of air left in their lungs, called *residual volume* (RV).

Breathing is so vital to life that the respiratory control center is housed in one of the most primitive parts of our brain, the medulla oblongata. This part of the brain is capable of continued functioning despite loss of consciousness, ensuring that critical functions like breathing are always maintained. The brain's respiratory center communicates with the diaphragm via the phrenic nerve. This allows the brain to either speed up or slow down our breathing. So even when we are sleeping or unconscious, as long as the brain stem's connection to the diaphragm via the phrenic nerve is intact, breathing continues.

One might envision that if we were designing this system, we might have little sensors that would tell the brain when oxygen levels in the blood were getting low. The brain could then send signals back to the lungs to tell them to breathe more quickly and deeply. The body's solution for this problem is even more complex. It includes a backup system housed in the brain, as well as input from peripheral receptors that monitor not only oxygen but carbon dioxide and pH levels in the blood as well. When carbon dioxide dissolves into the blood, it combines with water to become bicarbonate, which serves an important role in regulating the acid-base balance in the blood (measured in units of pH). The body is one highly orchestrated symphony of thousands of simultaneous chemical reactions, all finely tuned to optimal performance at a very specific pH: 7.4. A pH of 7.0 is perfectly neutral, with 7.4 being slightly alkaline. So when breathing alters the concentration of carbon dioxide in the blood by a significant amount, the pH in the blood also changes. Too much carbon dioxide and the blood becomes acidic. Too little and the blood becomes too alkaline, or basic.

We can think about the lungs like a conveyor belt, picking up oxygen and dropping off carbon dioxide with every breath. Chemoreceptors housed in the carotid artery monitor oxygen, carbon dioxide, and pH to determine how fast or slow breathing should occur. If all is functioning properly, then the body has enough oxygen and just the right amount of carbon dioxide to maintain a pH of 7.4. But if the system is perturbed, this conveyor belt really only has two options, to speed up or slow down. This system can handle "normal" perturbations such as exercise. When we exercise, we typically use more oxygen but also generate more carbon dioxide that we need to get rid of. So speeding up the conveyor belt helps with both problems.

What if, however, you want to take an airplane trip. Every time you board a flight, you inadvertently walk into an evolutionary blind spot. The interior of a plane is typically pressurized to the equivalent of roughly 6,000 to 8,000 feet above sea level. While the percentage of oxygen in inspired air is constant at various altitudes, the drop in total atmospheric pressure at higher altitudes results in a drop in the partial pressure of oxygen. At 8,000 feet, the partial pressure of oxygen is roughly 34 percent of what it is at sea level.[4] Partial pressure refers to the air pressure contribution from any single gas within a mixture of gases. This reduction in the partial pressure of oxygen reduces the driving pressure of oxygen into the blood, resulting in decreased oxygen content of the blood. The body responds by trying to breathe more, to speed up the conveyor belt. But unlike exercise, where oxygen demand and carbon dioxide generation more closely match each other, in this case speeding up the conveyor belt to deliver more oxygen also has the unfortunate consequence of ridding the body of too much carbon dioxide, thereby increasing blood pH.

If we reach higher elevations more slowly, the kidneys, which also play a key role in maintaining the body's pH balance, can over days to weeks bring the blood pH back into equilibrium. On the plane, however, the body settles on a compromise with suboptimal oxygenation but less severe acid-base disturbances than might otherwise occur. If we instead travel quickly to high altitude and stay there, the combination of low oxygen compounded by pH disturbances can lead to symptoms such as headaches, fatigue, and nausea—otherwise known as "acute mountain sickness."

As opposed to the effects we notice from this involuntary control over our breathing, conscious control over our breathing patterns, particularly slow, deep breathing, may also have profound effects on the rest of our body. Controlling one's breath to enhance health has been practiced by Eastern cultures for thousands of years. While the exact mechanisms are not well understood, slow breathing has the ability to alter brain activity and nerve signals going to other organs, such as the heart. Deep breathing exercises have been shown to lower heart rate, blood pressure, and even cortisol levels, which are a measure of the body's stress response. Slow breathing has well-documented effects on improving mood, reducing stress, and triggering a relaxation response. Slowing down the breath can also improve our attention span and even lower pain levels. Hence, the lungs not only provide life-giving oxygen and rid our bodies of potentially toxic carbon dioxide, the act of breathing itself contributes to our day-to-day sense of well-being.

Chapter 2

The Battle Within

YOUR LUNGS VERSUS THE WORLD

The lungs have a pretty big job to do. Taking in oxygen and expelling carbon dioxide is needed to sustain life, and it requires the lungs to circulate roughly 11,000 liters of air in and out daily. But that air often carries with it a host of other things: particulate matter from air pollution, smoke, noxious gases, and respiratory pathogens, including bacteria, viruses, and fungi. The lungs are in a constant battle against the outside world. They must limit collateral damage and exchange gas at the same time. How do they do it? The answer lies in a complex system of physical and immunologic safeguards. Understanding the lung's defense system helps us better understand the relationship between pollution, infections, and lung diseases.

The body's immune system is broken into two parts. The first is called *innate immunity*. If the lung's defense system were classified like the branches of the military, then innate immunity would be the marines, a versatile first-response team that provides nonspecific defenses. Innate immunity includes physical barriers in addition to specialized types of immune system cells that can attack foreign invaders. Physical barriers start right at the entry point, the nose. The complex branching structure of the nasal passages helps to trap particles before they ever reach the lungs. In addition, the cells that line the nose, sinuses, and much of the upper airways also create mucous secretions that help to trap particles. In fact, production of this gel-like substance is induced by harmful things like bacteria and cigarette smoke. Cilia, the tiny hairs that also line much of the respiratory tract, sit in a thin liquid layer, and a gel-like mucous layer sits on top of that. Like a tiny coordinated orchestra, the cilia beat in a synchronized fashion to create waves. This allows the cilia to propel the mucus, along with bacteria and other particles that have been trapped in the mucus, up the airways toward the mouth, where they can be coughed out or swallowed.

The nasal passages and sinuses serve a second crucial defense function: heating and humidifying the air before it gets to the lungs. Desiccation of the airways would significantly impair function of the ciliary escalator, increasing susceptibility to infection. Having just the right amount of liquid and mucus at a precise consistency is crucial for lung health. The genetic disorder cystic fibrosis results in severe lung damage and infection because the liquid layer is too thin and the mucous layer is too thick, resulting in a broken ciliary escalator.

To clear out the smaller particles that do land in the alveoli, the lungs rely primarily on innate immune cells called *alveolar macrophages*. For noninfectious particles, the alveolar macrophages not only clear them, but also help prevent unnecessary and potentially harmful further activation of the immune system. However, the lungs can't fully digest some nonbiological particles such as asbestos, silica, and coal dust. This can lead to chronic inflammation. These are just a few of the many potentially inhaled substances that, if present in high enough concentrations over long periods of time, can cause chronic lung disease.

Infectious agents can be recognized by the immune system because they carry specific markers called *pathogen-associated molecular patterns (PAMPs)*. Surfactant, which helps the lungs by reducing surface tension, can also bind to PAMPs on bacteria, viruses, and fungi, making it easier for alveolar macrophages to identify and digest them. PAMPs also stimulate airway epithelial cells to express chemicals that attract another cell type, neutrophils. Neutrophils are one of the most plentiful type of immune cell. They are highly attuned to killing PAMP-expressing microbes and are able to roam freely throughout the body to play a key role in fighting these foreign invaders.

The second branch of the lung's defense system is called *adaptive immunity*. This subset of the immune system is where our immune memory lives. Continuing with our military analogy, adaptive immunity can be thought of as special forces units. Components of adaptive immunity include highly specialized white blood cells, including B cells and T cells, that can develop immune responses to very specific pathogens. B cells make and secrete antibodies, also called *immunoglobulins*. Immunoglobulins defend us by binding to viruses and microbes, thereby inactivating them; they may sit on the surface of immune cells or be secreted. B cells mature within the bone marrow. Through random rearrangement of certain gene segments, a large repertoire of B cells is created that carries a huge variety of immunoglobulin surface receptors. Put together, this B cell army can theoretically bind almost any conceivable molecular target. These cells, however, may be short-lived unless they interact with a foreign "antigen" (*anti*body *gen*erator). Antigens are usually protein substances on the surfaces of cells, viruses, fungi, and bacteria, but they also include nonliving substances such as chemicals, toxins, drugs, or other foreign particles that induce an immune response from the body. After antigen exposure, memory B cells that are much longer-lived persist and can more quickly respond when challenged again by the same microbe. When activated, memory B cells divide into numerous plasma cells that can make large amounts of targeted antibodies when presented with a familiar microbe. This is the concept behind vaccinations.

T cells are another member of the adaptive immunity team. Among their multiple functions, T cells can directly kill infected host cells before viruses have had a chance to replicate. T cells also produce signal molecules that can help stimulate the innate immune system to destroy invading microbes. Further, T cells divide into "effector" T cells, which, when exposed to specific antigens, form a killing army targeted to those antigens. As with B cells, we also have long-lived memory T cells that can expand rapidly upon reexposure to specific antigens. Central to all of these immune system processes, however, is an elaborate system of checks and balances that involve both pro- and anti-inflammatory responses. This system helps the body to fight infection, but also regulates inflammation to limit collateral damage to the lung's delicate architecture.

The Lung Microbiome

When I started medical school, I was taught that the lungs in the healthy state are a sterile environment. We already knew that bacteria live on the skin, mouth, and gastrointestinal tract. But cultures from the lower airways of healthy individuals typically do not grow anything in the standard petri dish used by hospital laboratories, except bacteria known to live in the mouth, which traditionally have been viewed as sample contaminants. However, the development of molecular techniques that can identify bacteria or viruses based on identification of their genomic material reveals a much more interesting story.

To think that the lungs were free from bacteria was probably always a bit naive given that we've known that the mouth, nose, and throat harbor bacteria, and they are anatomically connected to the lungs. The lungs are also constantly bombarded with air and secretions coming from the upper airway. Now that we have very sensitive methods to detect microbes within the lungs, there has been significant debate in the academic community as to whether these microbes are "real." In other words, perhaps they just represent contamination from the sampling procedure or were washed into the lungs, but were essentially dead and not actually living within the lungs. One of the best analogies here is offered by Robert Dickson, an expert in this area, who compares the lungs to a tide pool. The community of animal life in the tide pool is determined by what washes in and out from the ocean, but we wouldn't say that the tide pool is devoid of life. In healthy lungs, it appears likely that the microbiome membership reflects the spillover from the upper airway but not active reproduction within the lungs themselves.[1] The clinical significance of these resident bacteria is still being investigated.

However, in patients with chronic lung diseases, we are learning a lot about the complexity of the organisms in the lungs and how it may contribute to human health and disease. We are finding that diseased lungs harbor a different set of bacteria compared with healthy lungs, even in diseases not previously thought to be caused by an infection. When the lung's defense mechanisms are impaired, new ecological niches develop that allow specific types of bacteria to grow. In other words, in diseased lungs, microenvironments develop within various regions promoting growth of specific bacteria uniquely suited to those conditions. Even for two people with the same chronic lung condition, there is significant variation in the type and amount of bacteria present, which may contribute to how well they do. Trying to understand the potential role of these bacteria is currently an active area of research.

Infections

We typically use the term *infection* to indicate that a microorganism is not just present but is also making us sick. There are a multitude of invaders that can and do attack the lungs on a regular basis. These include viral, bacterial, and fungal pathogens. When these infections cause symptoms right away, we call them "acute" infections. But other infections can be more insidious and take a while to cause symptoms. We call these infections "subacute" or "chronic" infections. It is worth mentioning that in the twenty-first century, we are increasingly using a wide range of medications to suppress the immune system for a variety of common conditions, leading to infections we had only rarely seen in humans previously. We use the term *opportunistic infections* to describe such infections in immunosuppressed patients.

Viral Infections

Some viruses primarily infect the respiratory tract, while in other cases the lungs become damaged as part of a more generalized attack on the body. I am going to focus on viruses that primarily infect the respiratory tract. Even within the respiratory tract, some viruses attack mostly the upper airway and throat, whereas others primarily invade the lower airways and sometimes the alveoli. Viral infections can also impact the resident bacterial flora of the lungs, particularly in people with underlying chronic lung conditions. Therefore, "primary" viral infections can lead to "secondary" bacterial infections. This has been commonly described with pneumonia caused by influenza viruses, where superimposed bacterial infection can significantly increase how sick a patient becomes.

One of the most frequent viral infections is the common cold, which may be caused by a large number of viruses, including rhinovirus, adenovirus, influenza virus, respiratory syncytial virus

(RSV), parainfluenza virus, and coronavirus. This is partly why we have no vaccine against the common cold. Other viruses known to invade the respiratory tract include the measles virus, enterovirus, hantavirus, the herpesviruses (including herpes simplex virus, Epstein-Barr virus, cytomegalovirus, and varicella-zoster virus), and the human immunodeficiency virus (HIV). Each of these viruses differ in their structure. For instance, adenoviruses are constructed from DNA. Coronaviruses are made of RNA. Some of these viruses only live in humans. Others, like coronaviruses, can be found in a wide variety of animals. Though they are rarely transmitted across species, there can be devastating consequences when they are. Some respiratory viruses can be found in secretions from the airways but also in urine, stool, tears, breast milk, and blood. For other respiratory viruses, such as the influenza virus, virus particles are found primarily in the respiratory tract.

The primary mode of transmission depends on the virus. For many respiratory viruses, large amounts of virus particles can be found in respiratory secretions, expelled into the air through sneezing, coughing, and breathing. Large spray droplets may land directly onto mucous membranes or contaminate objects facilitating viral transfer from the hands to the mouth, nose, or even eyes. While these larger droplets fall to the ground relatively quickly, smaller particles called *aerosols* may linger in the air for hours, traveling longer distances. For SARS-CoV-2, initial public health guidance focused on reducing droplet transmission through hand washing and social distancing, but mounting scientific evidence suggests that aerosols are a significant mode of transmission for SARS-CoV-2. This realization has refocused public health measures towards masks and improved ventilation.

Once a virus has access to cells lining the respiratory tract, it begins to invade. Many respiratory viruses have been detected in cells lining the nose, throat, and large airways. In the most severe cases, viruses can even be detected within cells lining the alveoli. When damage is isolated to the nose and throat, we experience symptoms of the common cold. Some viruses, such as herpes simplex virus, may cause shallow ulcers in the mouth and throat that can be quite painful. Infection of the bronchial tree leads to irritation resulting in cough. Inflammation in the smaller airways can make it difficult for air to pass. This may cause wheezing, particularly in young children.

One of the most common but concerning respiratory viruses for children is respiratory syncytial virus. RSV is the number one cause of lower respiratory tract infections among children in their first year of life and can lead to hospitalizations and even death. Some studies suggest that RSV infections occurring early in life may be associated with increased risk of developing asthma later in life, although children in these studies may already have had other risk factors for developing asthma.[2] Nearly all children become infected with RSV at some point. In adults, RSV can cause serious respiratory difficulties among immunocompromised individuals and those with underlying chronic lung disease.

Symptoms may be mild in some patients, but in others the impact of respiratory viral infection can be severe. Respiratory viruses can cause damage all the way down to the alveoli. When the alveoli become inflamed and fill with fluid, we can see this on a chest X-ray as a lung "infiltrate"—in other words, viral pneumonia. Influenza virus is an important cause of pneumonia, particularly in adults. However, other viruses, including RSV, adenovirus, parainfluenza virus, and varicella virus, can also cause pneumonia in healthy adults. Many people do not realize that the measles virus can also cause severe pneumonia, even among otherwise healthy individuals. The varicella-zoster virus, which causes chicken pox as a primary infection and shingles later in life due to reactivation, is another virus that can evolve into pneumonia. In fact, the likelihood of pneumonia with primary varicella-zoster virus infection is 25-fold higher among adults than in children.

Other respiratory viruses make curiously irregular appearances. In 1993, a young Navajo woman and her fiancé in New Mexico died suddenly from pneumonia, leaving behind an infant son. For two young, otherwise healthy people to die so suddenly from pneumonia is very unusual. Then others in the area, mostly also Navajo, experienced the same fate. Soon the Centers for Disease Control and Prevention (CDC) was brought in to investigate. CDC scientists ultimately traced the illnesses to a previously unknown hantavirus. As all other known hantaviruses were transmitted to people from rodents, CDC scientists set out on a colossal mission to capture nearly 1,700 rodents from the Four Corners region of the southwestern United States. They identified the deer mouse as the virus reservoir and named the new virus Sin Nombre virus (SNV). Researchers then scoured archived lung tissue from individuals who had previously died from unknown causes and discovered that a 38-year-old Utah man had died of SNV over 30 years earlier, in 1959. The 1993 cluster of cases was linked to a surge in the deer mouse population that year. While a handful of SNV infections are still reported annually, most, but not all, occur in the southwestern United States.

Diagnosis of viral infections of the respiratory tract has been revolutionized by the development of nucleic acid amplification testing. Although various types of such technologies are now available, larger clinical labs often use commercially available tests that can identify viruses based on their DNA or RNA signature. These tests can simultaneously screen for a large number of routine human viral pathogens from respiratory secretions, usually collected via a nasal swab. In my role as a pulmonologist at a large medical center, obtaining respiratory viral panels has become routine among patients with suspected respiratory viruses. We now have a much better sense of which viruses a patient is infected with than we did when I started my medical training in the 1990s.

Outside of prevention, we have limited treatment options for viral infections beyond general supportive care. For influenza, a series of antiviral drugs have been approved by the Food and Drug Administration (FDA). These drugs may shorten the course and severity of illness but work best when initiated within the first 48 hours after the onset of symptoms. For RSV, the antiviral medication ribavirin has been approved but has significant side effects that limit routine use. Antiviral medications to treat other specific viruses exist, but are typically reserved for those with severe infections or those who are immunocompromised. In general, such medications do not work as quickly or effectively as antibiotics do for bacterial infections.

Fortunately, vaccinations are available for certain viruses. This includes vaccines for measles, varicella-zoster (chicken pox vaccine for children and shingles vaccine for older adults), and influenza. Unfortunately, some viruses may have multiple strains circulating at one time. Rhinovirus, accounting for roughly 75 percent of colds in adults, has at least 160 different strains. These strains carry different proteins on their surface. Hence, designing a vaccine effective against all of these strains has proved to be very difficult. Fortunately, the illnesses caused by rhinovirus tend to be mild.

One vaccination program, however, has saved thousands of lives: the one for influenza. Influenza results in between 250,000 and 500,000 deaths globally every year. Significant resources are spent annually, forecasting which influenza strains will be most prevalent and developing new influenza vaccines. New influenza strains may be the result of subtle shifts ("antigenic drift") in the viral RNA that causes changes in the proteins encapsulating the virus, making previously developed antibodies less effective. Larger such shifts may occur for influenza when new genes encoding surface proteins are picked up from animals. This can happen, for instance, when animals become coinfected with a human and animal strain, allowing genetic material from the two strains to intermix. Antigenic shifts can lead to pandemics, as there is little to no existing immunity within the population. The vaccine-manufacturing systems we have in place for influenza are incredible in that we have the ability to manufacture new influenza vaccines every year, tailored to the strains believed most likely to be relevant in any given year. As we are all now well aware, developing new vaccines from scratch typically takes many years due to extensive safety and efficacy testing.

The COVID-19 vaccines aside, it is astounding how much resistance there is to vaccination, for influenza in particular. Like many practitioners, every year I hear the same litany of excuses:

"Last year I got the flu from the flu shot."

"I never get the flu."

"One year, I got vaccinated and still got the flu."

I try to make clear to my patients that these are all bad arguments. Just because you've never had the flu doesn't mean you're not susceptible. Further, many people say they have the "flu" when they really mean they have a bad cold, not influenza. Therefore, many don't understand just how serious influenza can be. While vaccination may lead to arm soreness or fatigue for a few days, such effects are nothing compared with influenza infection, which in severe cases can lead to respiratory failure and even death. This does not mean that more serious side effects never occur with vaccines. But they are rare, and overall the benefits far outweigh the risks. While the vaccine in any one year may not be perfect, it still offers some protection. I tell my patients that if they won't get vaccinated for themselves, they owe it to their loved ones. Even if you fare well with influenza, you might transmit it to someone who won't. The more people in a community that are vaccinated, the harder it is for the virus to spread, thereby offering better protection to the most vulnerable members of our society. This is what is meant by "herd immunity," which is thought to require at least 70 to 80 percent of a given population to have immunity to a specific virus. Having said that, too few people in the United States typically get the flu shot for us to ever achieve herd immunity.

SARS, MERS, and COVID-19

Coronaviruses with the potential to cause pandemics deserve special mention. MERS, SARS-CoV-1, and SARS-CoV-2 are all caused by coronaviruses. Coronaviruses have been recognized as a cause of the common cold for many years and in ordinary years cause anywhere between 4 and 15 percent of all annual respiratory infections. However, in recent years several novel coronaviruses have emerged as the cause of more severe respiratory disease. The first case of severe acute respiratory syndrome (SARS) is believed to have occurred in November 2002 in Foshan, China. By February 2003, over 300 cases had been reported with subsequent spread to other countries, including Vietnam and Canada. In April that year, the cause of SARS was identified as a coronavirus, labeled SARS-CoV-1. By July 2003, over 8,000 cases had been reported in 27 countries, resulting in over 700 deaths, but at that point no more infections were detected and the pandemic was declared over. Then in June of 2012, a man in Saudi Arabia died of pneumonia and renal failure. The novel coronavirus, Middle East respiratory syndrome coronavirus (MERS-CoV) was recovered from his respiratory secretions. A cluster of cases in a hospital in Jordan followed, later diagnosed as MERS. MERS continued to spread sporadically, with the most recent case in the United States identified in 2014.

Fast-forward to December 2019, when an outbreak of coronavirus was reported in Wuhan, China. Within a few weeks, the virus had spread throughout China. Almost immediately, the virus spread to other countries, including Italy, Spain, and the United States. Worldwide, by June 1, 2021, over 172 million

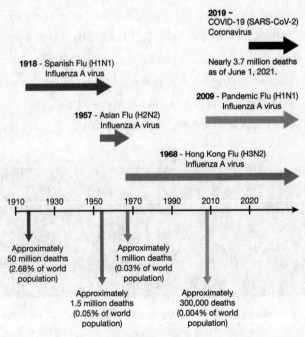

Adapted from a time line of pandemics since 1918.

individuals had been infected with SARS-CoV-2 and nearly 3.7 million had died. As with many other countries, in the United States we saw an initial surge of cases in late winter and early spring of 2020, a decline in cases during the warmer months, but a fierce second surge by fall and winter of 2020.

Some 50 million people died from the Spanish flu pandemic of 1918, roughly 2.7 percent of the world's population at that time. The Asian flu of 1957, Hong Kong flu of 1958, and H1N1 pandemic flu of 2009 were less devastating, resulting in roughly 1.5 million, 1 million, and 300,000 deaths, respectively. Few are now alive to remember the devastation of the 1918 pandemic, and many of us have been lulled into a sense of complacency.

Coronaviruses consist of a single strand of ribonucleic acid (RNA). The RNA sits in a spherical viral capsule with protruding spikes, giving the virus a "halo-like" or "corona" appearance under the microscope. These protein spikes allow the virus to latch onto human cells. The viral membrane fuses with the host cell membrane, such that the viral RNA can then enter the cell.

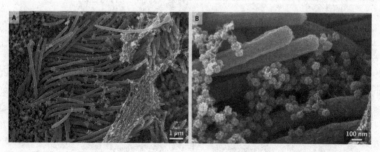

Respiratory cells 96 hours after infection with SARS-CoV-2, seen under an electron microscope. Virus particles can be seen coating the cilia of the respiratory cells underneath the mucous layer.

The viral RNA essentially hijacks the host cell and directs the host to create more copies of the virus.

Although the data are not conclusive, it is believed that the virus causing SARS-CoV-1 and MERS originated in bats and may have passed through civet cats in the former and dromedary camels in the latter before reaching humans. In some cases, spontaneous genetic mutations can allow the virus to invade and replicate within new hosts. In other instances, recombination with other viruses provides new genetic material that affords access to the new host. It is believed that SARS-CoV-1 arose from recombination.[3] The origin of the SARS-CoV-2 virus is still being debated.

Diagnostic tests for SARS-CoV-2 are commonly based on nucleic acid amplification technology, described earlier. How well the tests work, however, depends on where the sample is taken (upper versus lower respiratory tract) and operating characteristics of the test platform itself. Diagnostic tests that rely on viral antigen are generally less accurate than nucleic acid amplification technologies, but are also cheaper and easier to perform.

COVID-19, the clinical syndrome caused by SARS-CoV-2, is incredibly variable. Some patients are asymptomatic, though the exact percentage remains unclear. Various studies report that anywhere between 20 and 45 percent of infected individuals may be asymptomatic. However, asymptomatic does not necessarily mean no disease. Several studies have reported that a significant percentage of "asymptomatic" patients have some type of chest imaging abnormality. In some patients, the symptoms may simply not have manifested yet, as it is believed that the "incubation" period can be as long as 14 days following exposure.[4]

For those who do have symptoms, respiratory complaints including cough and shortness of breath are common, in addition to fever, body aches, and smell and taste disturbances. Several unusual manifestations have also been noted, including increased risk for blood clots that can occur anywhere in the body. We have also witnessed multisystem inflammatory syndrome in children (MIS-C), where multiple organ systems, including the heart, kidneys, lungs, brain, skin, eyes, and gut, can be affected due to an exaggerated immune response to the virus.

We are still trying to understand which patients are at greatest risk for severe disease with COVID-19. So far, older age, male sex, obesity, current smoking, and chronic conditions such as lung disease, cardiovascular disease, hypertension, diabetes, and cancer are among some of the risk factors. However, we have seen young, otherwise healthy individuals die as well, suggesting that no individual is without some risk.

Known complications from COVID-19 include kidney, liver, and heart injury in addition to excessive clot formation. However, one of the most dreaded complications is lung injury resulting in acute respiratory distress syndrome (ARDS). ARDS can be caused by many things, including severe infection and trauma. It essentially means that the lungs are severely inflamed, resulting in an inability to oxygenate the body. For medical personnel, ARDS has a technical definition that requires a low level of blood oxygen despite supplementation and chest X-ray evidence of pulmonary abnormalities on both sides of the lungs in the absence of another explanation.

One of the things we still don't know is what type of permanent lung injury patients who recover from COVID-19 infections will have. Among those who have come back in to see physicians for lung evaluation after infection, we are seeing patients complain about lingering cough, shortness of breath, chest pain, and fatigue. We don't fully understand whether these symptoms are due to damage to lung tissue, the airways, the blood vessels, breathing muscles, or even nerves. Another possibility is that lingering symptoms that appear respiratory in nature could also be due to damage to other organ systems, such as the heart. As lung function is not routinely measured in adults, we don't have much data on lung function on otherwise healthy individuals before they developed COVID-19. And even after patients have recovered from the acute infection, we do not yet have lung function testing data on large groups of individuals to indicate the severity of damage or rate of improvement. One small study of 57 patients demonstrated that at 30 days after discharge from the hospital, over half had abnormalities still present on chest computed tomography (CT) scans and 75 percent had lung function test abnormalities.[5]

By the end of 2020, it appeared that for the sickest patients, a steroid medication called dexamethasone and an antiviral medication, remdesivir, may be helpful. COVID-19 antibody-based therapies have also been given Emergency Use Authorization by the FDA to treat non-hospitalized, high-risk patients. By early 2021, nearly 3,000 clinical trials were either ongoing or completed and more than 70 vaccines were under investigation or approved. The first vaccines to receive government agency approval in the United States were mRNA vaccines utilizing novel technology. Traditionally, vaccines rely on eliciting an immune response through introduction of either viral proteins or live attenuated viruses. These novel SARS-CoV-2 vaccines deliver genetic code (messenger RNA) for building the coronavirus spike protein directly into human cells, causing them to make and release spike proteins, thereby provoking a response from the immune system. Data that has been released from clinical trials to date suggest efficacy rates exceeding 90 percent. Preliminary real-world data on the efficacy of the first two mRNA vaccines introduced in the United States also suggest 90 percent efficacy against SARS-CoV-2 infection.[6] To provide some perspective, the flu vaccine is typically 40 to 60 percent effective, whereas a three-dose regimen of inactivated polio vaccine is 99 to 100 percent effective. However, we still don't know how long immunity for any of the COVID-19 vaccines will last. It is also important to note that the first studies in children under 12 began in the spring of 2021 with early results anticipated by late summer or fall of 2021. We also still don't fully know to what extent existing and future mutations in the SARS-CoV-2 virus will affect vaccine efficacy. However, it is my firm belief that vaccines against SARS-CoV-2 offer the world our best hope to ending the pandemic quickly while sparing the greatest number of lives.

Bacterial Infections

Bacterial pneumonia is a major cause of illness among both children and adults. Worldwide, pneumonia is the leading cause of death among children under 5 and the sixth leading cause of death overall. Even in resource-rich countries, half of children younger than 5 years of age who develop pneumonia require hospitalization. Among adults, 30 percent of those who develop pneumonia require hospitalization. We divide bacterial pneumonia into two broad categories, community-acquired pneumonia (CAP) and hospital-acquired pneumonia (HAP), also sometimes called nosocomial pneumonia. The distinction is important because CAP can usually be treated with "empiric" antibiotics, meaning we take our best guess at the most likely bacterial cause to pick an appropriate antibiotic. HAP tends to be more serious. The microbes that cause HAP tend to be harder to treat and more resistant to antibiotics, so we do our best to identify the cause. We need to be more certain we are using the right antibiotic to reduce risk of treatment failure. This is not only to the benefit of the patient, but also to reduce unnecessary antibiotic use that may contribute to the global problem of bacterial resistance to antibiotics. As both the number of older individuals treated with immunosuppressive medications and the number of residents in chronic care facilities have increased, so has the complexity of treating bacterial pneumonia.

Bacterial pneumonias are thought to originate via aspiration of secretions from the nose and mouth. While we are awake, we do a pretty good job of protecting our airway. But when we sleep, we can aspirate small amounts of secretions from the throat. The mouth, nose, and throat of even healthy individuals are home to millions of bacteria. Some of these bacteria are considered part of our normal microbiome, while others carry "pathogenic" potential, meaning they can cause disease. Certain bacteria are common causes of more mild community-acquired pneumonia (sometimes called "walking pneumonia"). These include *Myco-*

plasma pneumoniae, Streptococcus pneumoniae, Chlamydia pneumoniae, and *Haemophilus influenzae* (not to be confused with the influenza virus). Other bacteria, such as *Staphylococcus aureus, Legionella pneumophila, Pseudomonas aeruginosa,* and certain bacteria referred to as "gram negative" (due to their lack of picking up a commonly used stain in the laboratory), tend to be more dangerous actors and may result in hospitalization.

In 1841, the ninth president of the United States, William Henry Harrison, lasted just a month in office before dying of pneumonia at the age of 68. Before the advent of antibiotics, William Osler described pneumonia as the "captain of the men of death" due to its high mortality rate, between 30 and 40 percent.[7] Today we are better able to treat pneumonia, but it can still be quite serious. The very young and the very old are at increased risk for poor outcomes with pneumonia, but so are other groups. Heavy alcohol consumption, for instance, is a risk factor for development of CAP due to impaired consciousness. Alcohol may also weaken the immune system. Smoking increases the risk of developing bacterial pneumonia, as do chronic lung conditions such as COPD and cystic fibrosis, due to lowering the lung's mechanical and immunologic defense shields.

Certain types of pneumonia are associated with unique exposures. The bacterium *Legionella* has been known to cause outbreaks when water supplies become contaminated. Legionnaires' disease got its name after a previously unknown strain of bacteria was identified as the cause of 182 cases of pneumonia among people attending a convention of the American Legion at the Bellevue-Stratford Hotel in Philadelphia in 1976.

Patients with bacterial pneumonia typically present with fever and respiratory symptoms, including cough, sputum production, shortness of breath, and chest pain. Occasionally, patients cough up blood. As noted, we call this hemoptysis. In older patients, symptoms may include a change in level of alertness, mood, or awareness of their surroundings.

In some patients, fluid may develop in the pleural space, the space outside the lungs but within the chest cavity. This fluid is called a *pleural effusion*. If we don't know the cause of an effusion, we typically try to sample the fluid with a procedure called a *thoracentesis*. If infected, the fluid needs to be drained to prevent complications; additional analysis of the fluid can also point us toward the cause of fluid buildup. For generations, medical residents have recited the mantra, "Never let the sun set on an untapped pleural effusion." As a medical resident, I spent many nights hunched over the bedside of patients to perform this procedure. Most commonly these occurred at 3 or 4 a.m., the only time that could be found on a call night. The attending physician would expect to have the results on morning rounds to guide management. Having said that, it is more common now for several suns to rise and set before effusions are tapped. We currently perform many more thoracenteses using ultrasound guidance as a scheduled procedure that can also provide information on the amount and characteristics of the fluid, which in some cases may even obviate the need to sample the fluid. However, if a significant amount of fluid is present and bacteria can be isolated from the fluid, it is called an *empyema*. Here we need to act more aggressively to drain the fluid and in some cases place a temporary tube to allow ongoing drainage for a period of time.

As with viral pneumonia, a chest X-ray is typically the first test ordered to establish the presence of an abnormality, but chest CT scans are more sensitive. For hospitalized patients in particular, we typically try to obtain sputum samples to determine which bacteria are present as well as their antibiotic sensitivity profiles. Unfortunately, patients can only cough up an adequate specimen about 40 percent of the time. For some bacteria, such as *Legionella*, the bacteria may shed particles into the urine that can be detected. Sometimes, particularly if the patient is not responding to antibiotics or we are unable to obtain a sputum sample, we may perform a bronchoscopy to obtain samples from the lower airways that can then be cultured for bacteria.

We choose antibiotics for CAP by targeting the most common organisms, such as *M. pneumoniae* and *H. influenzae*. For treatment of CAP that requires hospitalization, we tend to favor intravenous antibiotics to ensure that adequate levels of antibiotic are getting to the lungs as quickly as possible. However, treatment of patients with HAP and in particular ventilator-associated pneumonia (VAP) is more complicated because some of the organisms that cause these types of infections are more difficult to treat. Here we are more concerned about strains of *Staphylococcus aureus*, *Pseudomonas*, and other gram-negative bacteria that may be antibiotic resistant. For all patients, early initiation of antibiotics is believed to be important.

We currently have two primary vaccines for bacterial pneumonia in adults, both for *Streptococcus pneumoniae*. Here we specifically target individuals over the age of 65, in addition to those who are immunocompromised or have chronic conditions. As viral pneumonia caused by influenza can predispose to secondary bacterial infections, annual administration of influenza vaccine may also help to protect against bacterial infections.

Mycobacterial Infections

Mycobacteria are a type of bacterium worthy of special mention. Within the genus *Mycobacterium* are *M. tuberculosis* and a large number of nontuberculous mycobacteria (NTM). *M. tuberculosis* is well known as the cause of tuberculosis (TB). We sometimes forget that by the beginning of the nineteenth century, tuberculosis had killed roughly one in seven of all individuals who had ever lived. Referred to as the "white death," the disease was feared and so poorly understood that some doctors believed the condition was inherited. The belief that fresh air, high altitudes, and sunshine could be curative was instrumental in the development of such cities as Denver.

Although we now know much more about how the disease is transmitted and can be treated, the World Health Organization (WHO) estimated that as of 2020, roughly 2 billion people were still infected with TB, with numbers increasing by roughly 10 million persons annually.[8] TB is present in every country around the globe. Although it is true that countries such as South Africa and India have a greater prevalence of cases, in 2018 the United States still saw roughly 10,000 new cases. Despite ongoing efforts to combat this disease, TB remains the leading cause of death from infectious diseases worldwide and has been selected by the Bill and Melinda Gates Foundation as a key target disease for funding.

Tuberculosis is transmitted by inhaling infected respiratory droplets. Health care settings use a combination of negative-pressure rooms with high air exchange rates and UV lights to reduce risk of transmission. TB infection is broken into two phases. When a person first becomes infected, we call this "primary infection." Primary infection leads to pulmonary symptoms in roughly one-third of individuals, including fever and chest pain. However, many individuals experience no symptoms. The majority of individuals with intact immune systems are able to either clear the bacteria or contain them. If the bacteria are contained but not cleared, the infection enters a "latent" phase. During the latent phase, the individual experiences no symptoms, but the infection may reactivate at any time. For the small number of individuals who do not initially contain the disease, the infection may progress beyond the lungs to the rest of the body, particularly among those with poor immune systems.

"Latent" TB has classically been diagnosed with a skin test in which purified protein derivative (PPD) from the tuberculosis bacteria is injected into the skin. In infected individuals, swelling at the site (termed a "wheal") within 72 hours suggests the presence of latent TB. The interpretation of this test depends on clinical judgment as well as patient circumstances. Patients outside the United States often receive a TB vaccine called BCG, which if administered at birth provides at least some protection for children against the most severe forms of TB, but probably offers limited protection to adults against pulmonary TB. It is routinely used outside the United States due to the high prevalence of disease in certain countries. Previous BCG vaccination may impact interpretability of the TB skin test, although whether prior vaccination should be considered in the interpretation of the skin test is debated. Blood tests are now also available to identify TB infection. Though such tests can't distinguish between latent and active disease, the blood test is not affected by BCG vaccination status.

Reactivated TB represents the majority of clinical cases in the industrialized world. The most common symptoms are persistent cough, occasionally with blood. Patients also often have fever, night sweats, weight loss, and enlarged lymph nodes. With an initial infection, we often see evidence of infection in the middle and lower parts of the lungs. Reactivation TB, however, typically develops in the upper parts of the lungs and may lead to cavity formation within the lung tissue. If TB gets into the bloodstream, infection can deposit throughout the lungs and the rest of the body. Such widespread TB, termed "military" TB, can be quite dangerous.

TB can be difficult to treat because it is slow growing and drug resistance is increasing— a significant global public health concern. There are currently 10 drugs approved by the FDA for treatment of TB. Most regimens require multiple drugs taken for at least several months if not longer.

Nontuberculous mycobacterial infections represent another important problem. Roughly 50 species of NTM have been identified, with varying levels of potential to cause disease in humans. The presumed source of NTM infection in humans is the environment as opposed to the human-to-human transmission seen in TB. NTM can be found in both water and soil. In one study of 37 US patients with NTM infection, 46 percent of household water systems had at least one NTM species found in the patient. Use of indoor hot tubs and swimming pools are documented risk factors for development of NTM infection. While we don't know why, clinical NTM disease in the United States is more common in older women. The term "Lady Windermere syndrome," associated with NTM infection, was coined from Oscar Wilde's play *Lady Windermere's Fan*, in which the lead character actively suppresses a chronic cough. Underlying chronic lung disease such as cystic fibrosis and COPD also appear to be risk factors for clinically significant NTM infection.

Some NTM species are more likely to be contaminants in respiratory specimens due to their ubiquitous nature in the environment rather than actual infection. Hence, unlike TB, where a single positive sputum culture or bronchoscopic specimen is enough to establish a diagnosis, repeated isolation of a single species of NTM is typically preferred to increase diagnostic confidence. Also unlike TB, diagnosis of NTM does not necessarily require treatment. If symptoms and CT findings are mild and the patient is older and unable to tolerate therapy, we may choose to observe as opposed to treat. Treatment for NTM infection typically requires long-term treatment with multiple drugs that have significant side effect potential. Even then, treatment is not always successful. So for some patients, the treatment may be worse than the disease.

Fungal Infections

Mycoses is the medical term for fungal infections. Fungi are a group of microorganisms that include yeasts, molds, and even mushrooms. Fungal infections of the lungs are split into "endemic" and "opportunistic." Endemic fungal infections occur in certain locations where those organisms live in the environment. In North America, such organisms include *Coccidiodes*, which is found in the Southwest, and *Histoplasma* and *Blastomyces*, which are found in the Ohio and Mississippi River valleys. Infection typically occurs when fungal spores are inhaled from soil or water. Opportunistic infections are those we see primarily in immunocompromised hosts.

Symptoms and manifestations of these infections vary, depending on the species. Symptoms may be similar to viral and bacterial pneumonia, including cough and fever. However, for some mycoses, it is estimated that a significant percentage of primary infections never come to medical attention due to minimal or no symptoms. The fungi endemic to the United States can all cause not only acute pneumonia but also chronic infections. In some instances, these infections may also spread to other organs beyond the lungs. And in other cases, while the infection itself may have cleared, scarring in the lungs from prior infection persists. In Michigan, where I live, evidence of prior histoplasmosis infection is a very common finding on chest CT. While the remnants of prior infection in many cases are inconsequential, they can occasionally cause significant problems. With histoplasmosis in particular, the body's reaction can be so intense that the lymph nodes in the center of the chest enlarge and coalesce into a mass that can occasionally cause problems. One such patient of mine periodically coughs up what look like little rocks that we call "broncholiths." These are lymph nodes that have become so calcified that they occasionally erode into the airway.

Opportunistic fungal infections occur when fungi that typically do not cause human disease are able to cause clinical infection among immunocompromised hosts. Such fungi include *Cryptococcus*, *Candida*, *Aspergillus*, and *Mucor* species. In general, diagnosis depends on culture from respiratory secretions or blood antibody tests. Antifungal drugs are available, although some opportunistic fungal infections can be very difficult to treat. However, many times no treatment is needed for fungal pneumonia in otherwise healthy patients.

Chapter 3

Protecting Your Lungs for Life

Humans don't reach peak lung function until roughly 25 years of age. While this seems like a mere statement of fact, when we consider policies ranging from tobacco control to the proximity of schools to freeways, this simple statement has far-reaching impact. Normal lung development occurs in three stages: the fetal development period; growth during childhood and adolescence, when we achieve our best lifetime lung function in early adulthood; and a slow but inevitable decline in lung function as we age. For years, physicians ascribed to the notion that the majority of individuals start out their adult life with a "healthy" pair of lungs and that a subset, due to noxious exposures, experience more rapid declines in lung function that ultimately lead to diseases such as COPD. While we knew that factors such as prematurity and childhood respiratory infections could impact lung growth, we thought this was only relevant for a minority of the population.

Recently, however, the field of pulmonary medicine has been turned on its head with the discovery that roughly *one-half* of adults with COPD, the most common adult lung disease, *did not* experience accelerated decline in adulthood.[1] Instead, their lung function deficits were actually due to never having reached predicted normal levels of lung function as a young adult in the first place. This means that something went wrong during the first two phases of development for a much larger swath of the population than we had thought. It is estimated that well over 300 million persons in the world are living with COPD. Hence, it may not be only a tiny fraction of individuals who experience impaired lung development. The real number could be millions of such individuals.

If this is true, what exactly is going wrong, and why? There are a multitude of factors over a lifetime that could contribute to the development of lung disease. But pause with me for a moment to think about this another way. There are also a multitude of factors that contribute to our lung health. In other words, we need to think not only about factors that could cause us harm but also the factors that help us achieve and maintain our best possible lung function. Why don't we talk more about lung health?

To begin, unlike height, weight, and blood pressure, which are widely measured and tracked, lung function measurements are not performed on a routine basis during childhood. The first time I had my lung function measured was during pulmonary fellowship training in my early 30s, and even then it was for the purpose of understanding how the tests were performed. As a consequence, the majority of us have no idea how healthy or unhealthy our lungs are. There is no way to know what trajectory our lungs have had or what level of function would have been possible under ideal conditions.

For better or worse, the lungs also have a large amount of reserve capacity. This means they can sustain significant damage before we may notice that anything is wrong. It is only when something goes wrong that patients present to their physicians, and it is usually only then that physicians begin performing diagnostic testing.

Western physicians are trained to diagnose and treat disease. While disease prevention is certainly part of our education, the concept of actively promoting health is not something we talk about nearly enough. Patients are never referred to me, a pulmonary specialist, because they want to understand how to keep their lungs healthy. They are referred only if there is a suspicion of lung disease. Even our medical billing system is based on disease diagnosis codes. Contrast this to Eastern approaches to medicine, which consider health as a balanced state versus disease as an unbalanced state. The goal of Chinese medicine, for instance, is to maintain health by keeping the body in balance. Hence, the concept of health is not simply the absence of disease.

To be fair to Western medicine, it is only recently that data from research studies suggest that a wide degree of variation may exist with respect to lifetime lung function trajectories. It is also important to understand that from a health economics perspective, we typically order tests only if there is something obvious to do with that information. Otherwise testing is not considered cost-effective. Because so much is still not under-stood, it is not clear that we as medical practitioners would do anything different if, for instance, it was noted that a child's lung function trajectory was veering off course. This is because in most instances there would be no specific pill or therapy to recommend; the general recommendations promoting a healthy lifestyle remain the same for all patients.

However, it is crucial to understand that this is from the point of view of the physician and the health system. This may not rep-resent the viewpoint of an individual patient. What if there were specific behaviors you could adopt or harmful circumstances you could avoid that would provide you or your children the best possible chance of preserving lung health? Maybe you would make different everyday choices. The key here is arming your-self with information.

Protecting Lungs in the Womb

There are some simple things we can do to protect the lungs of unborn children, even as early as conception. But first we must understand when and how the lungs develop. The begin-nings of lungs are first detectable at around week 3 in the human embryo. This is known as the embryonic period. By week 5, two lung buds are evident. By week 8, the lung lobes begin to form, and by week 16, the airways complete their seemingly infinite branching. Between weeks 16 and 25 is when the alveoli, our gas exchange units, begin to develop. Amniotic fluid is essential for normal lung development at this stage. In the womb, the fetus "breathes" amniotic fluid, which mechanically stretches the developing lungs. Very low levels of amniotic fluid can disrupt fetal lung growth.

It is not until around week 20 of gestation that the alveolar cells begin to manufacture surfactant, a substance crucial for proper lung function and lung defense. However, the fully formed alveoli in their adult configuration are not present until roughly 5 weeks *after* delivery, and the alveoli continue to subdivide after birth. Recent data suggest that alveoli may continue to develop during childhood and adolescence.[2] This is important because some studies suggest that a subset of individuals with impaired lung function in early life may be able to "catch up" by the time they become young adults.[3] We still don't fully understand what allows some individuals to catch up and others not, but theoretically, factors that both contribute to and detract from lung growth could be just as important during childhood as they are in the womb.

Infants born prematurely are at risk for having inadequate surfactant, leading to respiratory distress syndrome (RDS), previously called hyaline membrane disease. Surfactant in immature lungs does not have the same chemical composition as surfactant in mature lungs, and its ability to lower surface tension to enable alveoli to open is not yet optimal. This is also where we begin to see sex differences in lung development. Male preterm infants are at significantly greater risk for RDS than female infants due to later initiation of surfactant production. Administration of steroids to pregnant mothers speeds fetal lung development and is generally administered to all pregnant women at 23 to 34 weeks of gestation who are at increased risk for preterm delivery within the next seven days.

Infants who experience RDS are at increased risk for a more chronic lung condition called *bronchopulmonary dysplasia* (*BPD*) that can involve scarring of both the airways and the alveoli. Prematurity and very low birth weight are also independent risk factors for BPD. Infants diagnosed with BPD, and even preterm infants who were not formally diagnosed with BPD, tend to have lower lung function when measured in adolescence or early adulthood.[4] It is difficult to speculate what the picture will look like for babies born today. The good news is that we know much more than we did 20 years ago about how to limit lung injury in preterm infants, but at the same time we also have technologies that now allow even younger infants to survive. Still, it is highly likely that the association between preterm birth, very low birth weight, and reduced pulmonary function will remain. The US preterm birth rate (12 per 100 live births) is higher than in similar countries such as Canada and Great Britain. Some have speculated that differences in rates of obesity, chronic health conditions, income disparity, unintended pregnancies, and higher rates of multiple gestation pregnancies related to assisted reproduction may all contribute to the higher rates of preterm births seen in the US.[5]

So what can we do to protect the lung health of unborn infants? A review of the available literature suggests there are factors that increase the odds of an infant being born with healthy lungs. But first, a quick word about data interpretation will help to put this discussion into context. Scientists evaluate the quality of data generated from studies based on the characteristics of the study design, the number of patients examined, and the number of studies conducted on a particular topic. All these factors influence the quality and weight of the evidence. Randomized controlled trials (RCTs) randomly assign either an intervention or a placebo to individuals so that other factors that could influence an outcome, such as age, weight, and eating habits, are evenly balanced between the two groups; in this way, any difference in outcome can be attributed to the intervention itself. Any other type of study that tries to look at associations between two factors in a group of individuals will almost certainly be subject to bias. If, for instance, you want to look at the association between drinking green tea and longevity, you might compare the life span of people who report drinking green tea versus those who don't. But the people who choose to drink green tea could have other factors that make them different from those who don't drink green tea. They may be more active or have healthier eating habits. What if there is an unidentified gene that both makes people like green tea and contributes to longevity? These other factors could also influence longevity, thereby introducing bias. So data derived outside of RCTs need to be viewed with a bit more skepticism.

In observational studies (not RCTs), many prenatal factors have been linked to reduced offspring lung health. Maternal hypertension, diabetes, obesity, and psychological stress have all been associated with wheezing episodes or development of asthma in childhood. Optimizing maternal physical and emotional health is the best way to optimize fetal lung health and overall fetal health. In 2017, globally fewer than two-thirds of pregnant women received the recommended four or more antenatal visits, and nearly 20 percent of women reported no health insurance prior to pregnancy.[6] To the extent that it is possible, establishing good prenatal care is the first step to ensuring a healthy pregnancy and healthy infant lungs. This also means, generally speaking, that medications required to keep mothers healthy will ultimately benefit the baby, excluding medications known to be unsafe in pregnancy. I have seen many women come into my office who have stopped all of their medications the second they found out they were pregnant. While decisions about starting or stopping specific medications during pregnancy should be discussed with a health care provider with expertise in obstetrics, an overarching guiding principle is that a healthy mom (including medications that are required for the maintenance of health) equals a healthy baby.

Though babies aren't actually "breathing" in the technical sense in the womb, maternal smoking is still damaging for developing lungs.[7] Globally, the prevalence of smoking during pregnancy has been reported to be as low as 5 percent in Sweden, Austria, and Switzerland and as high as 40 percent in Greece.[8] In the United States, roughly 20 percent of women report cigarette smoking during the three months before pregnancy; roughly 10 percent of women report cigarette smoking during the last three months of pregnancy.[9] Multiple observational studies have shown an increase in wheezing, respiratory illness, and asthma among children born to mothers who smoked during pregnancy. Longer-term studies show that even among children aged 8 to 12 years, lung function abnormalities still persisted among those whose mothers smoked during pregnancy.[10] Having said this, not all children exposed to smoke in utero will have impaired lung function. The timing, duration, and overall amount of smoke exposure likely play a role.

Animal studies suggest that it may be nicotine itself that is toxic to the fetal lung. There are many nicotine receptors within the human lung, and nicotine is known to cross the placenta. Animal lungs exposed to nicotine show enhanced collagen deposition that may impact how compliant (or not compliant in this case) the lungs are as well as how easily air flows through the bronchioles. Other data suggest that nicotine exposure during the period when the airways are developing (roughly 16 weeks gestation and beyond) may stimulate too much airway branching, leading to long, tortuous airways that impede airflow.[11]

If nicotine is indeed the bad actor that the data suggest, then electronic nicotine delivery devices (referred to as e-cigarettes from here onward) would theoretically pose similar risks to unborn infants. Use of e-cigarettes has recently exploded, in particular among teenagers and young adults. While we do not yet have long-term data on the lung function of children born to women who use e-cigarettes, the data we do have suggest that women should not be lulled into a false sense of security that switching to e-cigarettes during pregnancy is a "safe" option. In fact, e-cigarettes typically deliver as high or higher amounts of nicotine than conventional combustion cigarettes.[12]

Nicotine is a highly addictive substance, and some women may simply be unable to quit smoking completely. A randomized clinical trial demonstrated that vitamin C supplementation (500 milligrams a day) to pregnant smokers who were unable to quit smoking may prevent some of the effects of smoking on fetal respiratory health.[13] Newborns whose mothers had taken vitamin C demonstrated improved pulmonary function as compared to those whose mothers didn't. While these differences did not persist in the infants at the 1-year mark, infants of mothers in the vitamin C group still had significantly less wheezing during their first year of life than the offspring of mothers who took placebo. A second similar study found that several markers of pulmonary function at the age of 3 months were improved among infants with vitamin C–treated mothers as compared to placebo-treated mothers.[14] Incidentally, in several other observational studies, vitamin C (often taken along with vitamin E) was associated with lower risk for placental abruption and preterm birth among women who smoked.[15] While vitamin C is considered generally safe during pregnancy,[16] any nutritional supplementation during pregnancy should be discussed with the health care provider overseeing the pregnancy. Quitting smoking (if possible) is still the best approach to safeguard fetal lung health.

Beyond vitamin C, there is sparse data to suggest that other aspects of maternal diet impact the lung health of offspring, although maternal undernutrition clearly impacts fetal lung growth and development. Vitamin A is important for proper development of the airways and alveoli. Vitamin D aids with surfactant metabolism. Omega-3 fatty acids may also help protect the lungs of preterm infants. A Mediterranean diet high in fruits, vegetables, legumes, whole grains, fish, and nuts and low in meat and dairy products has multiple beneficial health effects for mother and baby, including reduced gestational diabetes, lower risk for allergic diseases, and potentially improved lung function in childhood.[17]

Characteristics of pregnancy and delivery, including pre-eclampsia, antibiotics during pregnancy, and even cesarean delivery, have in some studies been associated with increased risk of offspring asthma in childhood. A fairly large body of evidence links cesarean delivery to childhood asthma, allergic diseases, diabetes, and even inflammatory bowel disease. With any observational study, however, it is important to note that there may be things about infants born via cesarean section that also make them different from infants born via vaginal deliveries that could contribute to these associations.

One hypothesis that has been offered to explain the association between cesarean delivery and asthma has been coined the "bacterial baptism" of vaginal birth.[18] While most people probably don't realize it, vaginal delivery colonizes the baby with maternal vaginal and bowel bacteria. Cesarean delivery results in the infant being exposed to a different set of bacteria. Data do support differences in the gut microbiome of infants born via vaginal versus C-section delivery that persist months after delivery, although these differences disappear once food is introduced. The clinical significance of these early differences and the extent to which other factors such as use of antibiotics and breastfeeding could also be influencing these relationships are unclear right now. Because of the data, there has been increasing popularity in a practice called vaginal seeding, where the doctor swabs the vagina and then rubs the infant with those swabs after birth. At this point, however, we have very little data to support the effectiveness of this practice and some reason to think it could transfer harmful bacteria to the infant.

Protecting Lungs in Childhood

Given the many known health benefits of breastfeeding, it's not a surprise that the lungs should also benefit. Breastfeeding has been well established to reduce the incidence and severity of lower respiratory tract illness, which globally is a major cause of infant death.[19] Breastfeeding is also associated with lower risk for childhood asthma.[20]

Pneumonia kills over 2 million children worldwide every year, and lower respiratory tract infections in childhood have also been associated with reduced peak lung function and more rapid decline of lung function in adulthood.[21] Of all the causes of respiratory infections in children, respiratory syncytial virus (RSV) is among the most notorious. RSV infection in childhood has been associated with development of asthma and lung function abnormalities later in life.[22] As with all observational studies, it is not clear whether it is the virus itself that triggers the problem or whether viral infections are a marker of other abnormalities that predispose the infant to asthma. We do not yet have an RSV vaccine. However, childhood vaccinations play a central role in protecting children against respiratory infections in general.

Other viral infections, including rhinovirus, have also been associated with subsequent development of asthma.[23] Child-hood vaccinations that protect the respiratory tract in particular include vaccines against viral pathogens such as influenza, polio, measles, and varicella (chicken pox) in addition to bacterial pathogens such as *Streptococcus pneumoniae*, *Bordatella pertussis* (whooping cough), and *Haemophilus influenzae* type b. The data are clear: vaccination programs save millions of lives. And childhood vaccinations have the potential to protect children not only in the short term but also in the long term.

Severe malnutrition, seen more commonly in low- and middle-income countries, likely leads to smaller lungs and bodies in general. On the other hand, obesity is also problematic and has been associated with higher rates of asthma among children. As with pregnant mothers, a Mediterranean diet may promote lung health in children. Several studies have linked improved lung function in childhood and adolescence as well as lower prevalence of asthma to healthier diets, particularly those rich in fruits and vegetables.[24] Vitamin D may also be helpful. Vitamin D helps to maintain immune function and plays a role in lung development. Exclusively breastfed babies are at risk for low vitamin D levels, and supplementation is often recommended. For older children, obesity, inadequate consumption of fortified milk and dairy products, and low sun exposure in combination with light skin pigmentation are all risk factors for low vitamin D levels. (Milk is routinely fortified with vitamin D in the United States.)

To many, there seem to be more and more children with allergies of all kinds than there used to be. The types of bacteria and fungi that children are exposed to early in life may play a role. The "hygiene hypothesis" was originally generated as a potential explanation for why children raised in West Germany were found to have significantly higher rates of asthma and hay fever than those raised in Communist East Germany, despite higher air pollution in the east. Children who lived on farms in particular had lower rates of asthma and allergic diseases. The label "hygiene hypothesis" was born from a concern that an overly hygienic lifestyle and "sterile" home environment does not allow for adequate childhood exposure to microorganisms during childhood. For instance, long-term exposure to animal stables until the age of 5 has been associated with very low rates of asthma. While there is no clear link to personal cleanliness and allergic diseases, it may be that early exposures to a wide variety of microbes blunts the arm of the immune system responsible for allergic reactions. Incidentally, there is currently no strong evidence to suggest that probiotics reduce development or severity of allergic diseases.

Air pollution is another factor that can influence the lung health of children, yet many causes of air pollution fall below the radar of the general public. Air pollution can be caused by particulate matter—essentially dust and smoke particles in the air. Particulate matter comes from things like combustion of gasoline and wood, smokestacks, unpaved roads, and construction sites. Generally speaking, the smaller the particulate matter, the farther down into the lungs the particles will land. Air pollution can also be caused by gases such as nitrogen dioxide, sulfur dioxide, and carbon monoxide. The primary source of nitrogen dioxide pollution is combustion of fossil fuels, particularly from cars. Emissions from cars and power plants can also promote the formation of ozone. While ozone in the stratosphere is protective, it is a harmful air pollutant in the lower atmosphere near ground level. Ozone is toxic to the lungs, causing inflammation and even cell death.

Air pollution related to climate change, extreme weather events, and natural disasters such as wildfires are becoming real threats to human lung health. Hotter temperatures and drought both increase dust and particle pollution. Wildfires have become a major source of extremely high particle levels, noticeable even hundreds of miles from the fires themselves.

The data are clear that air pollution can negatively impact lung growth in children.[25] Air pollution exposure can also make asthma symptoms much worse for children, leading to flare-ups called *exacerbations*. For some children, exacerbations may lead to emergency department visits and hospitalization.[26]

So what exactly can we do about this? Many of us can't control the city we live in, but we may be able to control whether we live near a highway. Residential proximity to a highway has been associated with poor lung growth and lower lung function due to traffic-related air pollution. Interestingly, one study showed that children who moved to places with cleaner air experienced an increase in lung growth, whereas children who moved to more polluted areas experienced declines in lung growth. The American Lung Association creates an annual "State of the Air" report that grades air quality in the United States by zip code. The American Lung Association's Stand Up for Clean Air initiative also offers expanded guidance on how we can all help combat air pollution and reduce our own exposure. This includes things like widespread adoption of electric vehicles, using electric-powered as opposed to gas-powered lawn care equipment, avoiding outdoor exercise on bad air quality days or near high-traffic areas, and reducing vehicle emissions around schools through anti-idling policies.

Air pollution can also vary significantly on a daily basis. AirNow.gov allows you to look up the Air Quality Index in your area at any given time. On unhealthy air quality days, your best bet is to keep yourself and your children indoors if possible, with doors, windows, and fireplace dampers shut. Air cleaning devices with HEPA filters can provide additional protection. Unfortunately, if you must spend time outside, ordinary masks are not that helpful for filtering the smaller, more dangerous particles. An N-95 mask is required to filter the smallest particles, but such masks have become difficult to obtain and often do not come in sizes appropriate for children. When driving on unhealthy air days, roll up your windows and operate the recirculate setting for your vehicle's ventilation system.

Air pollution can also come from within the home. Sources of indoor air pollution include asbestos, building and paint products, cleaning supplies, mold, radon, residential wood burning, and secondhand smoke. One strategy to mitigate exposure is to use "low-VOC" (volatile organic compound) paints, which are now readily available. If you are installing new carpet, request that it be aired out before installation. Make sure you have working carbon monoxide detectors in your home. All homes should be tested at some point for radon, which is a naturally occurring substance that is a decay product of uranium. Radon is the second leading cause of lung cancer. Radon has been found at elevated levels in homes in every state, so the only way to know is to test. Radon mitigation systems can be installed if this is a problem in your home. For individuals with allergies to dust mites, which can exacerbate asthma, keeping home humidity low and replacing carpets with hard surface flooring can help.

An often overlooked source of indoor air pollution is residential wood-burning stoves. Solid fuels, including wood and coal used for cooking and heating in developing countries, are known to cause significant lung damage and predispose women and children, in particular, to the development of COPD. We tend not to think of "cooking over an open fire" to be of relevance in developed countries. However, many homes in North America, for instance, still use wood-burning fires in the winter. I grew up with a wood-burning stove in the home for winter heating, which was quite commonplace in Idaho. Emissions from wood smoke can not only exacerbate asthma, but also lead to long-term lung function impairments. If switching to natural gas, for instance, is not an option, consider upgrading to a clean burning device if possible. The Environmental Protection Agency (EPA) adopted new, stricter standards, so look for devices that meet the 2020 standards. Some communities have put in place woodstove change-out programs. Newer woodstove models feature improved safety and efficiency.

The youth tobacco epidemic is one of the biggest public health crises of our time, outside of the COVID-19 pandemic. The rising popularity of e-cigarettes among young people is one of the biggest drivers of increased use. The 2018 National

Youth Tobacco Survey reported a 78 percent increase in the use of e-cigarettes among high school students. By 2019, nearly one-third of American high schoolers and 10 percent of middle schoolers reported e-cigarette use.[27] Children use tobacco products for a wide variety of reasons, but most concerning is tobacco industry marketing of flavored products aimed at youth. One survey found that 43 percent of young people who ever used e-cigarettes tried them because of appealing flavors.[28] As a result of federal government inaction, e-cigarettes have been on the market in the United States with very little regulation. While it became illegal to sell e-cigarettes to children younger than 18 in 2016, in 2017, the FDA issued a guidance (directive) saying that the manufacturers of e-cigarettes, including the flavored ones that especially appeal to children, could keep those products on the market without FDA review until 2022. In May 2019, however, in a lawsuit brought by a group of organizations including the American Lung Association, American Academy of Pediatrics, and the American Heart Association, the court ruled that the FDA had acted illegally by granting that five-year deferral. As a result, in January 2020, the FDA changed its rules to require that all companies with e-cigarette products that wished to stay on the market file product review applications by September 2020. All such applications that were filed are currently under review by the FDA, with final decisions due by fall 2021. Research suggests that whether flavored products remain on the market will determine the true impact of this federal oversight with respect to e-cigarette use among youth.

The long-term effects of using conventional cigarettes are clear: increased risk for COPD, cardiovascular disease, and cancer, particularly lung cancer. The health effects of e-cigarettes have not been as well studied. E-cigarettes contain liquid that is heated to produce a vapor the user inhales. The components typically include nicotine, propylene glycol or glycerol, flavorings (with more than 7,000 available), and a myriad of other compounds, including metals such as tin, lead, nickel, chromium manganese, and arsenic. Other compounds that have also been detected in e-cigarette liquid include acetaldehyde, acrolein, and formaldehyde.

Here's what we do know about potential health effects. E-cigarettes are highly addictive. Depending on the amount and type of product used, vaping can deliver similar or even more amounts of nicotine with average use patterns as compared to conventional cigarettes. Despite marketing claims that e-cigarettes may be used to wean an individual from conventional cigarettes, the National Academies of Science, Engineering, and Medicine have concluded that if youths use an e-cigarette, they are at increased risk of using conventional cigarettes. Even more concerning, nicotine use in youth may have long-lasting effects on attention, learning, and memory.[29]

There are also reasons to be concerned about the impact of e-cigarettes on the lungs. Lab research shows that chronic nicotine exposure alone may cause airway disease.[30] E-cigarette liquid can impair the function of the cilia on the respiratory epithelial cells that play a crucial role in lung defense. Some of the other components of vaping liquid are known to cause cell death and lung scarring. Acrolein, for instance, is used to kill weeds and may cause lung cancer.[31] While we don't have a lot of long-term data, particularly among adolescents, recent data in adults suggest that e-cigarettes may increase risk for developing respiratory disease.[32] Secondhand emissions from e-cigarettes are theoretically equally concerning, carrying the majority of the same compounds.

Perhaps the best-known potential health hazard of vaping is EVALI, which stands for e-cigarette or vaping product use-associated lung injury. EVALI was first recognized in the summer of 2019. Since then, several thousand cases have been reported in the United States alone, with 68 deaths as of February 2020. Fortunately, the case count has since declined. Vitamin E acetate in the vaping liquid was identified as a possible culprit, but we still don't know if there are other chemicals in vaping liquid that could be responsible for the lung injury seen in some of the cases. Vitamin E acetate had been used more commonly in e-cigarettes containing tetrahydrocannabinol (THC), the main psychoactive component of cannabis (marijuana). While the initial scare is over, the potential for vaping to cause immediate harm to the lungs is now clear. It is also impossible to know when or if another compound could be added to vaping liquid that could lead to the level of danger we saw with the first EVALI outbreak.

The best medicine is prevention. US federal legislation passed in 2019 raised the minimum age of sale for tobacco products, including e-cigarettes, to 21, although we still see significant variation in the level of regional enforcement. When should we start talking to our children about tobacco products? While it is never too early, middle school is a good time to initiate these conversations. At this age, children are still receptive to advice from their parents. This is also the age where exposure to friends who use e-cigarettes begins to increase. It is important for parents to realize that vaping can also be very easy to hide. E-cigarettes don't leave the characteristic scent of tobacco, and vaping devices may look like common objects, such as a pen or flash drive. More information can be found through the American Lung Association (lung. org) on how to talk to your children about these complex issues.

For children and adolescents that are already using tobacco products, free programs and even apps are available to aid with smoking cessation. Talking with a child's pediatrician is another good first step. Teens are different from adults, and unfortunately, methods that may be helpful for adults may not be effective for youth, so specialized approaches may be needed. Varenicline, trade name Chantix, has been proven beneficial in helping adults to quit, but a recent study in teens did not demonstrate efficacy. Hence, it is now only indicated for individuals over the age of 16. [33]

We must also not forget the effects of secondhand tobacco smoke. Roughly 40 percent of US children aged 3 to 11 years are exposed to secondhand smoke, but the tobacco industry has sought to undermine research reporting on ill effects of this type of exposure. [34] Data from the European Union show that three out of five smokers allow smoking in their homes. The composition of secondhand smoke is nearly identical to that of firsthand smoke. Secondhand smoke causes serious health problems in children, including increased risk for sudden infant death syndrome and asthma exacerbations. Recent evidence suggests that heavy maternal smoking may be associated with reduced peak lung function and accelerated lung function decline in adulthood. [35] Children exposed to secondhand smoke also develop more frequent respiratory and ear infections. Parents can help to protect their children by not allowing anyone to smoke in or near the home, car, or child's day care center. Secondhand smoke can also infiltrate multiunit dwellings through vents and cracks in walls and floors. Some communities have laws that apply to secondhand smoke in multiunit housing.

Smoke from marijuana has many of the same toxins and carcinogens as tobacco smoke. Marijuana is also smoked differently. Deeper inhalations combined with breath holds increase tar exposure. Secondhand marijuana smoke is essentially the same as directly inhaled marijuana smoke. Whether marijuana is burned in a joint, vaped through an e-cigarette device, or dabbed (inhalation of flash-vaporized cannabis concentrate), concerns for damage to the respiratory tract exist. Smoking marijuana can damage the respiratory epithelium, leading to cough, wheezing, and phlegm production. As many marijuana smokers also smoke tobacco, the effects of each are difficult to distinguish. However, over the long term, the case against smoked marijuana versus tobacco is less strong. While marijuana use can clearly cause cough and sputum production, results from longitudinal studies are mixed with respect to long-term effects of marijuana alone on lung function or risk of lung cancer.[36]

Protecting Lungs in Adulthood

All the factors relevant to protecting the lungs in childhood are still important in adulthood. This includes limiting exposure to air pollution and obtaining recommended vaccinations to reduce risk for respiratory infections. While it's important not to start smoking, unfortunately 90 percent of all smokers start before age 18. This means that the most relevant message about smoking in adulthood is about quitting. In adults, long-term cigarette use is clearly linked to accelerated lung function decline, development of COPD, and increased risk for lung cancer. Most people don't realize that chronic tobacco smoke exposure may cause a wide range of lung diseases. One needn't smoke for 20-plus years to do significant damage. I have seen devastating consequences from smoking among even very young adults. The potential for tobacco to damage the lungs over a period of just several years should not be underestimated. Results from research are mixed as to whether e-cigarette use in adults improves quit rates from conventional cigarettes. The FDA has not approved e-cigarettes as a quit smoking aid. The bottom line is to stay away from inhaled tobacco products. If you are using, the most important thing you can do for your health is to quit.

The next thing you can do to improve your lung health is to ensure that you're breathing clean air. As with children, avoiding air pollution in our communities and in our homes is vital. For adults there are several other considerations worth discussing, both at home and in the workplace. Cleaning products often contain chemicals harmful to the lungs. Volatile organic compounds (VOCs), ammonia, and bleach can all irritate the airways. Never mix bleach or any bleach-containing product with any cleaner containing ammonia. The gaseous chlorine or hypochlorous acid created from this combination can cause significant breathing problems and even death. Ideally, choose cleaning products that do not contain (or that have reduced amounts of) VOCs, fragrances, and flammable ingredients. While the European Union restrictions on chemicals used in household products tend to be stricter than regulations in the United States, you can now refer to the EPA's list of cleaning products that meet their new "Safer Choice" requirements.

Another factor for adults to think about is protecting their lungs at work. Roughly 15 percent of all COPD cases in Western societies have been attributed to occupational vapor, gas, dust, or fume exposure, particularly in the mining, textile, and farming sectors.[37] Certain compounds known to cause lung disease include asbestos, silica dust, and coal mine dust. Other compounds, however, like aluminum, graphite, barium, and iron, can also cause lung disease. A wide variety of occupations are at risk for unclean air. This list includes, but is not limited to, farmers, factory workers, woodworkers, construction workers, painters, cleaners, taxi drivers, and hairdressers. Hairdressers, for instance, may be exposed to volatile organic compounds found in styling product propellants. Other potentially harmful alcohols are widely used in beauty products. A recent study found that airborne pollutants at work can increase your risk of developing COPD by 22 percent.[38] Secondhand tobacco smoke exposure in the workplace is another major issue for certain workers. This includes individuals in repair and maintenance, transportation, and entertainment sectors.[39] It is difficult to protect such workers short of tobacco-free policies.

There are lurking dangers even in office settings that we don't typically think of as being sources of air pollution exposure. For instance, printers and photocopiers release particles of a size that some studies in mice suggest can cause lung injury. Several cases of significant lung disease in humans have been reported in association with photocopier toner dust exposure, as well as chest X-ray changes and wheezing among individuals with longer-term exposures.[40] Spills should be handled carefully, and the use of regular vacuum cleaners should be avoided. Wiping solid surfaces with a wet paper towel or rag is a safer option to avoid kicking up dust.

Other ways to ensure clean air at work include keeping air vents open and substituting the use of hazardous materials with nontoxic alternatives. Regular maintenance to make sure ventilation systems are working properly and wearing protective gear as appropriate can also reduce risk.

Another common discussion I have with patients revolves around mold or mildew in the home or office building. Mold exists everywhere. No indoor space is mold free. However, excess moisture from flooding or inadequate exhaust of bathrooms and kitchens can promote increased mold growth. Significant mold exposure can worsen preexisting lung conditions such as asthma as well as potentially increase the risk of developing asthma in children.[41]

Still, there is not a lot of evidence to support more serious health risks among healthy individuals. Rarely, some molds, such as *Aspergillus*, can cause infections among immunocompromised individuals, although in my experience the majority of such mold infections occur even in the absence of exposure to obvious mold growth, suggesting that they may not have been preventable. However, if you are going to attempt cleaning up mold, the CDC recommends wearing an N-95 respirator. In some instances, the safest route is professional remediation. The Occupational Safety and Health Administration (OSHA) offers a technical guide to investigating mold problems in the workplace. The EPA also offers an indoor air quality building education and assessment model that may be valuable for facility managers, and trade organizations for specific professions may offer additional guidance.

Beyond protecting air quality, what other lung protective measures can you take? There are many reasons to exercise, but maintaining fitness levels in young adulthood may improve lung capacity in later adulthood. We know that aerobic exercise, such as walking, swimming, and jogging, improves circulation and lowers resting heart rate and blood pressure. Exercise likely also benefits the lungs. Studies show that aerobic exercise interventions can improve lung function in the short term. This is most likely because exercise strengthens the respiratory muscles and improves chest wall mechanics. However, exercise may also have long-term benefits for lung health.

In the National Institutes of Health (NIH)–sponsored study Coronary Artery Risk Development in Young Adults (CARDIA), data were collected on teens and young adults aged 18 to 30. These individuals were then followed for 20 years. What the researchers found was that for every additional minute an individual could walk on a graded treadmill test at the first assessment, the less lung function they lost over the 20-year follow-up period.[42] More specifically, the treadmill test used in this study consisted of nine 2-minute stages on the treadmill of increasing difficulty: from 3 miles per hour at a 2 percent grade all the way up to 5.6 miles per hour at a 25 percent grade. (Very steep!) Men and women with the lowest fitness levels could only exercise roughly 9 minutes and 6 minutes, respectively, whereas some individuals with the highest fitness levels were able to go the full 18 minutes. Individuals who sustained or increased their treadmill test time over 20 years of follow-up preserved their lung function better than those who experienced a decline in their treadmill test time. This suggests that having a base level of fitness at an early age is good, but so is maintaining or even increasing that fitness level over time. While experts recommend 150 minutes of aerobic activity a week to optimize heart health, we still don't know the exact amount of exercise needed to optimize lung health over a lifetime.

We also don't fully understand how exercise might protect the lungs. Inflammation levels in young adults have been associated with losing lung function more quickly. One possibility is that over the course of years, exercise helps lower inflammation levels in the body,[43] thereby limiting the impact of the repeated insults the lungs experience over time. So there are many reasons why aerobic exercise may be good for the lungs. It's never too early to start, but it's also never too late. We often put patients with even advanced lung disease through guided exercise programs called *pulmonary rehabilitation* that include aerobic exercise.

Patients often ask me whether various types of breathing exercises will help their lungs. We do know that in addition to the diaphragm, several upper body muscles, including the pectoralis major, trapezius, and intercostal muscles, termed accessory muscles of respiration, also help you breathe. Upper body resistance training that strengthens these muscles may make breathing easier, particularly for patients with chronic lung disease. It is probably not the lungs themselves that are changing, but rather our body's ability to more efficiently move air in and out of the lungs that improves with this type of exercise. Pulmonary rehabilitation programs designed to help patients with lung disease also typically incorporate upper body strength training.

Another type of breathing exercise that has been examined is called "inspiratory muscle training." This is done by breathing through a device specifically designed to make it harder to breathe, thereby "exercising" the breathing muscles. The consensus is that this is more beneficial for patients who have respiratory muscle weakness to begin with and probably not beneficial for the general population. Even among wind instrument musicians and singers, who use their respiratory muscles more than most, studies are mixed with respect to whether such individuals have better lung function than the average population.

While we've already covered the connection between diet and lung growth, in adulthood the issue is how we can best preserve lung function and reduce our risk for lung cancer and chronic lung disease. There is weak evidence to support a role for vitamins A, C, D, and E in slowing lung function decline in adulthood, but very little in the way of data from randomized, placebo-controlled trials. There is one RCT that suggests that vitamin D supplementation may benefit lung function among current and former smokers, particularly those who have vitamin D deficiency or those with asthma and COPD.[44] Population-based studies have shown preservation of lung function and reduced lung cancer risks with diets high in fruits and vegetables. Again, a Mediterranean-style diet high in fruits, vegetables, whole grains, and healthy fats and low in red meat has been linked to a multitude of health benefits beyond the lungs.

The summary? Don't smoke, don't vape, and if you are doing either, quit. Make sure you and your children have received recommended vaccinations. Be conscious of chemicals you are using in the home and at work as well as particles and gases in your environment. If there is a strong odor, investigate it. If you are cleaning anything that can kick up dust into the air or generate aerosols, think about how to reduce your exposure, and when in doubt, wear a mask that can filter small particles. Pay attention to your environment, and if the air quality index suggests an unhealthy air day, stay indoors when possible. Eat your fruits and vegetables, and if you aren't exercising regularly, now is the perfect time to start.

If you are experiencing chronic cough, sputum production, wheezing, and breathlessness, these symptoms are not normal. Talk to your health care provider about them and ask for a spirometry test. It is difficult to know anything with certainty without obtaining a spirometry test to measure how well your lungs are functioning. Spirometry is also not as sensitive for early lung disease, so further investigation with CT imaging may be required in some cases. As with just about any health problem, knowing earlier gives you and your health care provider the opportunity to intervene if there are modifiable factors contributing to lung problems, thus reducing the risk of further lung damage. I have witnessed too many patients who come to me with advanced lung destruction where our treatment options are limited. Don't wait.

Chapter 4

How Pulmonologists Think

THE SCIENCE AND ART OF
DIAGNOSING LUNG DISEASES

Going to see a physician, any physician, can be an intimidating experience. Let's be honest. Where else is it socially acceptable for a stranger to ask you to take your clothes off and then interrogate you with a bunch of personal questions? Of course, for those of us who work in health care, this is routine, but it reminds me a bit of the classic Hans Christian Andersen story "The Emperor's New Clothes." If we behave as if this is a perfectly normal thing to do, then maybe everyone will believe that it is. But I've also been the examinee, and I am well aware how anxiety provoking such experiences can be.

The experience that has forever shaped my understanding of being a patient was the 10 weeks I spent confined to the 9th floor of Von Voigtlander Women's Hospital in Ann Arbor, just steps away from my own office at the University of Michigan Hospital. I had been in Seoul, Korea, to deliver a lecture, 26 weeks into my pregnancy. I awoke in my hotel room with unexplained bleeding. I rushed to return to the same hospital where I had given a lecture earlier that afternoon. After a few days, my husband and I decided (against medical advice) to take a calculated risk for me to fly back to Michigan. I was rehospitalized within hours of my return, where I would remain until my son was born, at just under 36 weeks. Thankfully, he is now a rambunctious first grader. Not only did I develop an appreciation for the mental fortitude required to endure a prolonged hospitalization, but I also now know the loneliness that only illness imparts. But I was also incredibly fortunate. As a physician, I know how to speak the language and was able to advocate for myself and my unborn son. I know that this isn't a luxury that most people have, so I want to give you an inside perspective into a pulmonologist's way of thinking, so that you, too, can best advocate for yourself and your loved ones.

As a lung specialist, and in particular one who works at an academic institution, the majority of my patients have lengthy stories to tell. They walk into my office carrying with them a suitcase full of prior health care experiences that we must, together, unpack. I'm not speaking only metaphorically. Before the advent of electronic medical records, people really would show up to my office with a suitcase filled with records. In some instances, my review of these prior experiences led to solid answers. In other instances, they provided at least partial leads. In this way, my job as a physician is both detective and judge.

First I need to hear all the evidence. This is where the patient tells me their story. Then I need to inspect all the evidence. This is where I examine not only the patient, but also any medical records that may accompany them. Next I weigh the evidence, taking into account not only what's been written but also how credible I believe the source to be. Depending on the complexity of the case, in many instances I will want to review the physical evidence myself, not just reports of the evidence. Finally, I decide what additional testing is needed in order for me to render the best opinion I am capable of making.

If we are lucky, I will be confident in the diagnosis. There are many patients for whom the diagnosis is straightforward, and we may be able to help them feel better within a relatively few number of visits. In other cases, however, I am very honest with the patient that based on all the assembled information, I can be confident that the condition isn't X, but it still could be Y or Z. This is where patient conversations are so crucial to the decision-making process. Here is where what matters most to the patient will help to guide the path we take. In some cases, there are things that I must recommend very strongly. In other cases, I will ask my patients, "What keeps you up at night? Will having this additional information allay those concerns?" These are the kinds of questions that help me decide how far we should go with further diagnostic testing and what level of certainty we need to pursue.

Early in my medical school training, diagnoses were presented as clear-cut, black and white. I came to believe that if I just knew which tests to order, the diagnosis would be obvious. That this turned out not to be true was perhaps one of the greatest disappointments of my early medical training. No matter how many books I read, no matter how many lectures I attended or patients I saw, in some cases the final answer would remain elusive.

Unlike other organs, such as the skin or even the kidneys or liver, the lungs are not easily accessed for large biopsies. Cutting the lung can cause air leaks. Another challenge we face is that there is no easy, routine blood test that provides any insights regarding lung health. We have routine blood tests that tell us about kidney and liver function. For heart disease, blood pressure is a test done every time a patient goes to the doctor's office, and cholesterol screening is common. As a fellow pulmonologist, Dr. Ravi Kalhan, constantly reminds me, "We have no cholesterol of the lung." We have no objective measures of lung health that are checked in the course of routine medical care.

The lung can silently accumulate scars from repeated injuries over the span of years, and often only late in the course of disease does the lung become so damaged that the injury becomes evident. At this point, trying to understand by what mechanism this injury occurred can be very difficult. While certain types of lung function and CT scan abnormalities are more "characteristic," in some cases, severe scarring from a variety of causes can end up looking the same. This is like being asked to examine a crime scene years after the crime occurred. So it is not uncommon for me to be left with some degree of uncertainty, even after every test that could possibly be done has been run.

I say all of this to explain what lung physicians are up against. Yes, there are common problems for which the treatment plan is quickly apparent. But as a lung doctor, I have learned to live in the gray. Given so much uncertainty surrounding pulmonary diagnoses, we as chest physicians have developed systems to rely on one another's expertise. Diagnosis of certain scarring conditions we call interstitial lung diseases presents a particular challenge. Working at a large academic medical center, I am privileged to be able to confer on difficult cases with very skilled colleagues. We routinely meet with physicians in radiology and pathology to review cases, discuss diagnoses, and form treatment plans. Medicine has a long tradition of such case conferences. Tumor boards have been in existence for many years, allowing surgeons, pathologists, radiologists, and oncologists to all review cases and as a group solidify diagnoses and treatment plans. As a discipline, we have learned that together we are greater than the sum of our parts.

Several years ago, a young woman came into my office, having recently moved to Michigan to be closer to family who could help care for her. She had been diagnosed with a very rare, progressive lung disease that almost exclusively affects women: lymphangioleiomyomatosis (LAM). LAM causes destructive cysts to form within the lungs and is a disorder that I consult on frequently. She came to me to be started on the therapy she was told she needed, an immunosuppressive medication that has demonstrated efficacy for LAM. She had also been told she might need a lung transplant. When I first examined her CT scan, I felt uneasy about the diagnosis. The pattern of cysts didn't look consistent with the diagnosis. I discussed her case with our team, who instead favored a diagnosis of another type of interstitial lung disease, pulmonary Langerhans cell histiocytosis (PLCH), which also can cause cysts. This disorder can be associated with smoking, for which she did have a distant history. What can be confusing about the CT findings for this alternative diagnosis, however, is that while the CT scan may initially show cysts and little nodules, over time the nodules can begin to disappear from the CT, thereby making the diagnosis more obscure, particularly if the patient had stopped smoking.

I brought her back into the office to discuss next steps. Lung disease had upended her entire life. She needed certainty. She needed to know as much as possible about what her future might hold. Hence, for her, the right decision was to undergo surgical biopsy to firmly establish the diagnosis by examining the lung tissue. Indeed, the biopsy results were consistent with PLCH and not LAM. The difference in prognosis between the two diseases is significant. PLCH tends not to progress if the patient stops smoking. LAM typically is progressive. While we still had a lung disease to manage, securing a diagnosis for her allowed her to plan her life. For my part, I felt good knowing we had done the right thing for her. But getting to a diagnosis for some patients can be a complex process.

The Medical Interview

Even with our incredible advances in technology, obtaining an accurate medical history is still key to making an accurate diagnosis. Traditionally, the medical interview for all physicians is quite structured. This includes the history of the present illness together with the patient's past medical history, including any prior diagnoses and surgeries. We create a list of current medications, specifying any allergies to medications. We also typically ask about the patient's social history, which includes occupations, tobacco and alcohol use, and travel history, as well as any family history of medical problems. Finally, we perform a review of systems, where we ask about symptoms from all major organ systems that may not have come up earlier in the interview.

The primary respiratory symptoms lung physicians will ask about include shortness of breath and cough. Shortness of breath, or dyspnea as lung doctors like to call it, is a complicated sensation. In reality, it is poorly understood. And besides pulmonary conditions, cardiac, metabolic, and neuromuscular disorders can also cause dyspnea. Dyspnea is also tricky to assess because human beings avoid discomfort. So if an activity makes someone short of breath, they will often simply stop doing it. Hence, when asked if they are short of breath, some patients will answer "no" without providing a completely accurate picture of their respiratory health. For instance, a patient may deny shortness of breath, but upon further questioning tell me that they used to walk the golf course but now need to use a cart. These are the kinds of details I need.

Time course is also important. A change in symptoms over time suggests that whatever the problem is, it's getting better or worse. Dyspnea that is sudden in onset might suggest a collapsed lung or blood clot to the lung. I once interviewed a patient who could tell me the exact day and time when his dyspnea started, two years earlier when he'd fallen off a ladder. This led me to look for a paralyzed diaphragm, which in his case was caused by neck injury from the fall. The phrenic nerve takes off from spinal nerve roots at the level of the 3rd, 4th, and 5th vertebrae in the neck and hence is at risk for damage with neck injuries. Shortness of breath that occurs only with certain exposures, such as dusts, molds, and perfumes, or with exercise can be seen in asthma. Breathlessness that wakes a patient from sleep can occur from heart failure, but also from pooling of respiratory secretions. Breathlessness that occurs only when lying down, the supine position, points to some type of neuromuscular dysfunction.

Cough is another important pulmonary symptom. For most of us, coughing is associated with upper respiratory tract infections and is short lived. Cough that lasts longer can be related to things like postnasal drip, asthma, and heartburn. Certain types of medications, most notoriously a class of antihypertensive medications called *ACE inhibitors*, can also cause a cough. Physicians typically want to know not only how long the cough has been going on but also whether it is productive of mucus, as certain types of conditions are more likely to be associated with mucus production. Coughing up blood, hemoptysis, can occur with certain types of infections, but it warrants further evaluation if it persists. Hemoptysis can be significant in cancer and a host of rarer conditions.

Respiratory health begins in the womb. Maternal smoking as well as environmental tobacco smoke exposure during childhood increase the risk for reduced lung function later in adulthood.[1] Premature birth is associated with other types of respiratory complications that can persist into adulthood. Severe pneumonias can also cause certain types of scarring that may cause lung problems later in life. Further, there are other types of problems, like asthma, that may actually begin in childhood and then wax and wane later into adulthood. Interestingly, while as children boys are more likely to have asthma, they also tend to outgrow it as they reach puberty. After puberty, girls are more likely to have asthma, such that adult asthma is roughly 1.5 times more common in women than in men.[2]

Chest physicians always ask about certain types of exposures. Tobacco and more recently electronic cigarettes and vaping are clearly important, but there is a huge laundry list of lung diseases caused by very specific types of exposures. Pneumoconiosis is caused by dust deposition into the lung. Asbestos, coal dust, and silica are among the most notorious culprits. Another type of lung injury pattern, hypersensitivity pneumonitis (HP), can be seen with repeated inhalation and sensitization to antigens, which are molecules, often proteins but sometimes chemicals, that elicit a very specific type of immune response. The list of compounds that can potentially cause HP if inhaled regularly is nearly endless. Types of HP include farmer's lung, bird fancier's lung, cheese worker's lung, malt worker's lung, and woodworker's lung, just to name a few. Almost every pulmonologist will tell you that they have at least one patient who has HP due to a pet bird, but the patient refuses to give the bird up. Such is the love of some patients for their birds.

Another potential hazard pulmonologists are leery of is hot tubs. They can be problematic, particularly if poorly maintained or poorly ventilated. Several years ago, a new patient came into my office describing shortness of breath for about a year. After extensively interviewing him as well as reviewing his CT scan and lung biopsies, we felt confident that he was suffering from "hot tub lung." He explained to me that due to his arthritis, he frequently used his hot tub, which was in his basement. Hot tub lung is a form of HP caused by a class of bacteria called *nontuberculous mycobacteria* (NTM) that can grow in hot tub water. Repeated exposure to the antigens on the surface of the bacteria elicits a response from the immune system leading to lung disease. After several extensive discussions, the patient made clear that he could not bear to give up the hot tub. The compromise we landed on was that he would move his hot tub from the basement to outside his home to improve the ventilation. Once he did this, his breathing began to improve.

Finally, travel history is another important piece of the medical interview. Certain infectious diseases are more common in certain parts of the world. Tuberculosis, for example, is more common in India, China, Southeast Asia, and South Africa. There are also certain infectious respiratory diseases that are endemic to certain parts of the United States. When one of my uncles moved to Tucson, he developed a pneumonia that simply wasn't getting better with a standard course of antibiotics. A chest physician at the University of Arizona diagnosed him with valley fever, which is caused by the fungus *Coccidioides*. When people inhale the fungal spores that are found in soil, they can contract pneumonia. In healthy patients, the infection often resolves eventually without treatment, but all patients need to be closely monitored to ensure resolution. Antifungal therapies are available for patients who need treatment. As there are numerous infections endemic to various parts of the world, travel history is an essential part of the medical interview.

The Physical Exam

Modern-day physicians are not as adept at the physical exam as our predecessors were. Traditionally, the two required skills for examining the lungs are percussion and auscultation. Percussion is the art of tapping on the body and using the resulting sound to aid with diagnosis. Its utility was first discovered in 1761 by Leopold Auenbrugger, an Austrian physician who had noted that his father tapped wine casks to ascertain the amount of wine left. He extended the application of this technique to tapping on the human body, noting how the sound changes when percussing hollow versus solid organs.[3] Today, percussion is performed by placing one finger over the organ to be percussed while striking it with a finger from the other hand. Over a pneumothorax, the note is hyperresonant, whereas over a fluid accumulation in the lung or pneumonia, the sound is dull. When I began my career as a pulmonologist, it was quite commonplace to percuss the lung to identify where a needle should be placed to drain fluid from around the lung (thoracentesis). While medical students today are still taught to percuss the lungs, modern techniques such as ultrasound that can rapidly and accurately identify fluid around the lung are being increasingly employed.

Auscultation is the art of listening to the lungs with a stethoscope, which owes its origins to a French physician, René Laënnec. Laënnec invented the stethoscope in 1816 after watching children transmit sound signals to each other using a long piece of wood.[4] Normal lung sounds are thought to arise from turbulent airflow within the larger bronchi. A lung that becomes consolidated (as in pneumonia) leads to higher-pitched "bronchial" breath sounds. It is presumed that these sounds originate from the central airways with exaggerated transmission to the chest wall. Fluid that accumulates around the lung (known as a pleural effusion) tends to diminish breath sounds. Other types of sounds we listen for are rales, also called "crackles," which are thought to be caused by explosive openings of small airways that had been closed. Crackles are commonly heard in the presence of heart failure, which causes fluid to accumulate within the alveoli; these are sometimes called "wet" crackles due to their coarser sound. Pulmonary fibrosis is also a common cause of crackles, sometimes called "dry" crackles due to their finer sound. Dry crackles have been likened to the sound of Velcro opening. Wheezing is another sound that is commonly recognized. These are high-pitched sounds sometimes present in obstructive lung diseases such as asthma. Finally, *rhonchi*, sometimes called low-pitched wheezes, are a rattling sound thought to be due to fluid in the airways. There are several websites where you can listen to all of these sounds for yourself.

None of these skills, however, substitute for simply watching a patient breathe. I can spot some lung problems from across the room. Breathing should be easy, with roughly 12 to 20 breaths occurring in 1 minute in the average adult. Faster breathing may indicate distress. A patient struggling to breathe will sometimes bend over and use their arms to brace against their legs or on another surface to optimize the mechanics of breathing. Some patients may have a slightly blue tinge to their lips, suggesting low levels of oxygen. Other patients may slightly purse their lips as they breathe out, a maneuver that can help to open up the lower airways. Pursed lip breathing may be helpful particularly in obstructive diseases to keep smaller airways open during exhalation to release trapped air.

The body may provide other clues to the presence of lung disease. For example, bulbous enlargement of the ends of the fingers can be seen in certain types of lung diseases, such as scarring conditions of the lung. We call this clubbing. This distinctive abnormality can develop within as little as two weeks. Lung cancers can cause all sorts of abnormalities, including hoarse voice, muscle wasting, swollen lymph nodes, enlarged liver, and skin discoloration. So it can be important to examine the entire body, even when lung disease is the primary concern.

Pulmonary Function Testing

Pulmonary function testing is arguably the most important tool pulmonary physicians have for making accurate diagnoses and quantifying disease severity. While there were some prior cruder attempts, the first major advance in this area was made in the early 1800s by a physician and medical assessor for the Britannia Life Assurance Company named John Hutchinson.[5] Patients blew into a tube connected to the cavity of a calibrated bell inverted in water that would lift up out of the water proportionate to the volume of exhaled air. Although not the first to report this volume of air, he did give it its eloquent current name, "vital capacity," or the capacity for life. At the time, however, the invention really never caught on. After Hutchinson died, the practice of measuring lung function fell out of favor until the advent of the twentieth century, when forces outside of medicine made the ability to measure lung function suddenly relevant: World War I aviators began experiencing breathing difficulties flying at high altitudes; commercial manufacturing led to an increase in industrial lung diseases; and a boost in cigarette consumption heightened recognition of emphysema.

With further study, physicians began to realize that several common respiratory disorders, including asthma and emphysema, were not simply a problem of vital capacity, but rather the rate at which that air could be blown out. Lung diseases in which air is trapped inside the lungs are referred to as "obstructive" lung diseases. In 1947, the French physicians Robert Tiffeneau and André Pinelli introduced the concept of FEV_1, the forced expiratory volume in 1 second, arguing that the most important part of the vital capacity occurred in the first second. Today this is one of the most important parameters we look at on spirometry, although now we have electronic spirometers that calculate FEV_1 by measuring the speed of airflow using ultrasonic transducers. The data are fed into a computer such that the volume of exhaled air can be plotted against time, as can be seen in the following figure.

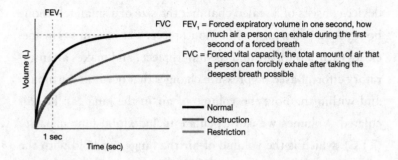

Spirometry patterns help diagnose lung disease. A plot of time versus the exhaled volume of air shows a normal exhalation pattern versus what is seen in patients with obstruction (such as asthma or COPD), where exhalation time is prolonged, or in restriction (such as pulmonary fibrosis), where total lung volumes are reduced.

We see obstructive spirometric patterns in diseases like asthma and emphysema. For such patients, it takes a very long time to breathe all of their air out compared with individuals without lung disease. A reduction in the ratio between FEV_1 and the amount that can be breathed out with a forced exhalation (forced vital capacity, FVC) indicates the presence of obstruction. FEV_1 itself helps us determine the severity of airflow obstruction. The lower the value, the worse the obstruction. If FEV_1 and FVC are both reduced but the ratio is normal, this is suggestive of a restrictive defect that can be associated with conditions such as pulmonary fibrosis. Formulas allow us to determine how close a patient's lung function comes to values that would be predicted based on factors such as sex and height.

Another modern tool we use for measuring lung function is the plethysmograph, informally called the "body box." This device consists of a sealed chamber the size of a small telephone booth equipped with a single mouthpiece. The patient sits inside, closes their mouth around the mouthpiece, and makes an inspiratory effort. Based on pressure changes that occur at the mouth and within the box, the volume of air in the lung can be calculated. Volumes we can calculate include total lung capacity (TLC), which is the volume of air the lungs can hold with the biggest breath, and residual volume (RV), the volume of air still left in the lungs after the patient has forcefully expelled all the air they can. TLC can be too large, for instance in patients who have emphysema and have lost their elastic recoil and develop air trapping; here often the residual volume also increases due to trapped air at the end of the breath. TLC can also be too small from interstitial lung diseases that can cause scarring, where elastic recoil is too high. Disorders of the chest wall that cause restriction can also cause low TLC, as can diaphragmatic dysfunction.

Another type of measurement frequently performed in pulmonary function labs is something called "diffusing capacity," more formally diffusing capacity of the lung for carbon monoxide (DLCO). To measure DLCO, the patient breathes a very small known amount of carbon monoxide. The change in concentration of carbon monoxide between the inspired and expired gas is a good surrogate measure of the capillary surface area available for gas exchange. I sometimes explain to my patients that spirometry helps us to understand how well the lung behaves as a bellows to move air, whereas DLCO tells us about how well gases are being transferred between the lung and the blood. While it is intended to assess the lung, I once diagnosed a woman with a gastrointestinal bleed based on a low DLCO. In her case, a low red blood cell count caused a significant and sudden reduction in measured gas transfer. After the anemia was treated, her DLCO returned to normal.

We have a variety of tests that help us to understand exercise capacity and the extent to which lung disease may interfere with that capacity. Perhaps the simplest and most widely used is something called the *6-minute walk test*. Here we examine not only how far a patient can walk, but also whether supplemental oxygen is needed by tracking blood oxygen levels via a device called a *pulse oximeter*. On the other end of the spectrum is a test called *cardiopulmonary exercise testing* that typically involves a patient either cycling a bike or walking on a treadmill; the lungs and heart are monitored closely during this test to help physicians understand whether exercise impairment is related to lung impairment, heart impairment, or something else.

Imaging

Imaging has significantly advanced the field of pulmonary medicine. Within six months of William Roentgen announcing his discovery of X-rays in 1895, battlefield physicians were using them to aid detection of bullets in wounded soldiers. Since then, our understanding of the benefits and risks of X-rays has increased exponentially. The basic principle is that X-rays are a form of electromagnetic radiation, similar to light. However, X-rays have much higher energy, allowing them to pass through objects like the body.

Traditionally, X-rays were detected on film. Black areas occur where X-rays expose the film, and whiter areas appear where travel of the X-rays to the film has been reduced by soft tissue and bone. While the detector used to be actual film, now digital sensors are used. When I was in training, all imaging studies for a single patient were kept in one, very large envelope or "film jacket" that floated between various floors of the hospital, depending on who needed to access it. My very first morning of internship, I was sent by my senior resident to the basement of the hospital to locate "the jacket" for the patient I was to present on morning rounds. The pressure interns experience on rounds is intense, particularly in July, the first month of internship. Like a rat running through a maze for the first time, I blindly sped through the basement corridors in a desperate hunt for the films. Half an hour and a few tears later, I finally located it. I don't even remember now what the films showed. What I do know is that somewhere toward the end of my pulmonary fellowship, digital imaging that could be accessed from any computer in the hospital arrived. Hallelujah! Now we can access films from anywhere, we can more easily transfer images from other institutions, and we can easily magnify images to examine specific areas of interest in greater detail.

In their simplest form, chest X-rays are the most widely available type of imaging that chest physicians have access to. It is still the first imaging procedure that many patients will receive. Such "films" typically include a lateral (side) view and a postero-anterior (PA) view, so called because the film or digital detector is in front of the patient and the X-ray source behind the patient. The chest is actually really difficult to image because there are such different tissue densities represented between the soft lungs and the denser tissues in the center of the chest, including the heart. This posed a greater problem with traditional film but is easier to manage with digital imaging.

Chest X-rays can be very informative, providing clinicians information about the presence of pneumonia as well as fluid in the lung (pulmonary edema) or around it (pleural effusion). Pneumothoraces can also be detected on chest X-rays, and we may even be able to identify lung cancers on chest X-rays. Because it is human nature to hone in on the most obvious abnormality while potentially missing something else more subtle but still important, radiologists approach chest X-ray interpretation in a very systematic way, methodically examining every structure. Chest X-rays remain an important and easily accessible first pass for chest physicians to identify abnormalities.

While chest X-rays allow us to look at the lungs from the front and the side, CT scans also give us slices through the middle, providing significantly more information. CT scanners are shaped like a large doughnut with a sliding table that carries the patient through the middle of the scanner. Inside the metal casing of the doughnut is a rotating circular frame with an X-ray tube mounted on one side and a detector on the other. The fan-shaped X-ray beam moves through the patient and is collected on the detector. The entire frame rotates around the patient; during each rotation, roughly a thousand images are taken that are then reconstructed by a computer to provide a cross-sectional picture of the body, typically capturing between 1 and 10 millimeters of body thickness per picture.

Chest physicians can learn a lot from CT scans, including the type and extent of abnormalities present in the lungs. It is not uncommon to identify a pneumonia on CT that was not well seen on X-ray. The lungs may have a moth-eaten appearance in the case of emphysema. We may see air trapping that is characteristic of small airway disease, seen in asthma. We may also see that some parts of the lung are hazy due to inflammation. We sometimes call this "ground glass," which means an area of lung has increased density (it is more white on CT scan), but not so dense that it obscures the underlying structures. Various types of scarring pattern can be seen that can indicate specific types of interstitial lung disease. Other types of abnormalities include enlarged lymph nodes, holes in the lung, or fluid around the lung. Using intravenous (IV) contrast, we can also image the pulmonary circulation, allowing us to identify blood clots. In the end, however, radiologists are interpreters of shadows. They may be able to point to a diagnosis or a group of diagnoses, but often cannot provide absolute certainty.

We also have a variety of other imaging tests used in specific circumstances. These include ultrasound, which may show how much fluid is present around the lung and where best to insert a needle to drain pleural fluid. V/Q scans rely on a combination of two radioactive tracers, one inhaled to identify areas of the lung that are well ventilated (V) and the other injected into the blood to show which areas of the lung are getting the most blood flow (Q, coming from the French word *quantité*, for "quantity or amount"). This test is often used for surgical planning. Although V/Q scans are much harder to interpret, we sometimes choose them over chest CT scans to identify clots if we are concerned about the potential to harm the kidneys associated with contrast dye. Magnetic resonance imaging (MRI) is used much more rarely for the lung. MRI technology is based on the identification of protons, most notably in water. The normal lung has very little water, making MRI somewhat less useful than CT to map lung structures, although techniques are being researched that may make MRI useful in evaluating certain aspects of lung disease. Finally, positron-emission tomography (PET) scans use radioactively labeled glucose tracer to identify cells that are rapidly dividing to help determine the presence of cancer.

Bronchoscopy

Bronchoscopy allows us to guide a fiber-optic camera through the nose or mouth down into the lungs to evaluate the airways and take samples. The diameter of the bronchoscope is roughly 5 to 6 millimeters, so we really can't get too far out into the airways with the camera itself. But we can rinse the lungs with saline (called a *bronchoalveolar lavage*) and via a suction channel sample the fluid to identify, for instance, causes of infection. We can also examine the types of lung cells collected, which may give us clues as to the type of inflammation present. We can pass tiny biopsy forceps through the scope to sample lung tissue.

However, biopsy samples obtained via bronchoscopy are quite small and therefore more diagnostically limited than surgical biopsy, where much larger pieces of lung tissue can be obtained. A newer technique using a cryoprobe can be used to make the specimen larger, but the risk of bleeding may also be higher. In the past few years, advanced three-dimensional guidance systems that map the lungs in real time have become available that allow us to more accurately direct the biopsy forceps to sample a tumor, for instance. Sometimes we will use CT guidance to pass a needle through the chest wall into the lung to take a biopsy, but the risk for pneumothorax tends to be greater with this type of procedure. We also have the ability to use ultrasound-guided bronchoscopy (endobronchial ultrasound bronchoscopy, or EBUS) to guide a needle into the lymph nodes surrounding the airways to sample some of the cells, most commonly to look for malignancy.

No test, however, is perfect, and they all must be combined with clinical acumen and experience. I once received a call from a friend that an abnormality had been picked up on her chest CT scan. Her pulmonologist was initially concerned about cancer, but the PET scan they ordered did not show increased uptake, suggesting benign behavior. However, review of prior scans suggested that the abnormality had in fact been there for a while and was slowly getting larger. Slow-growing lesions can be difficult to evaluate because they may not necessarily show increased uptake on a PET scan, as we typically see in cancer. Based on discussions about her case at our tumor board conference, the decision was made to move forward with biopsy

via three-dimensionally guided bronchoscopy. The biopsy con-
firmed cancer, and she subsequently underwent successful surgical resection. The bottom line is that no matter how perfectly
executed, diagnostic tests are only as good as the physicians
interpreting them. Patients need both high-quality tests and
experienced physicians who can put any single test into the
greater context of the patient's entire clinical picture.

Chapter 5

A Short Guide to Chronic Lung Diseases

The diagnosis of lung disease is part art and part science, like the rest of medicine. The complexities of the human body are nearly infinite, and therefore unknowable, even by the most astute clinicians. My most trusted pulmonary textbook is roughly 2,000 pages long, and there are still patients I have seen whose disease is not fully contained within those pages. The goal of this chapter is to provide an overview of the major categories of chronic lung diseases. This is the basic framework from which all pulmonary physicians begin.

Asthma

Asthma is one of the most common respiratory diseases today. Roughly one in 13 people have asthma, with children being affected more than adults. The prevalence of asthma has been increasing since the 1950s, and we don't fully understand why.

Asthma is an inflammatory disease of the airways. For a long time, asthma was thought to be driven primarily by allergic inflammation, involving the part of the immune system that reacts to specific allergens. This typically means an increase in specialized white blood cells called *eosinophils* and a specific class of immunoglobulins known as IgE. However, we now understand that not all patients with asthma have allergic inflammation.

So why are there so many people with asthma now? One theory, called the hygiene hypothesis, is that improvements in hygiene have led to a decrease in overall microbial exposure early in life, which in turn has altered the development of the human immune system toward allergic diseases. Another theory is that changes in home environments, like increased insulation and carpeting, along with more time spent indoors, have led to increased exposure to allergens such as dust mites. Other theories suggest that increased environmental air pollution or decreased physical activity could also play a role. No theories are conclusive, and all of these factors have been implicated. Whatever the reason, asthma now affects more than 25 million Americans and over 300 million individuals worldwide.

Even more alarming, according to the US Department of Health and Human Services, Blacks are three times more likely to die from asthma-related causes than whites. Black children have a death rate 10 times that of non-Hispanic white children, and Black women are 20 percent more likely to have asthma than non-Hispanic whites. While the exact cause for increased severity of asthma among Blacks is not well understood, these data point to the need for early identification and treatment of asthma among Black children in particular.

Clinical Presentation and Diagnosis

Due to chronic airway inflammation, patients with asthma experience wheezing, shortness of breath, chest tightness, and cough. For some patients, symptoms may become worse at night. Others may do fine for a period of time until exposed to specific triggers. Common triggers for asthma symptoms include exercise, cold air, and inhaled allergens such as dust mites, animal hair, or pollen. When patients have severe, more prolonged flare-ups requiring frequent use of short-acting bronchodilator medication (such as albuterol) and oral or injectable steroids, we call this an asthma exacerbation.

While often thought of as a disease that begins in childhood, the course of asthma over a lifetime can be quite variable. Boys tend to have more asthma in childhood than girls, but tend to grow out of it during puberty. By adulthood, more women have asthma than men. While asthma may begin in middle to late adulthood, and I have certainly seen this, a rigorous evaluation of other conditions, including cardiac disease, must be performed, given the increased likelihood of other chronic conditions with aging.

Diagnosis is based on the presence of typical symptoms, compatible pulmonary function testing, and exclusion of other diagnoses. Pulmonary function tests may show airflow obstruction. If so, we generally like to see that obstruction resolves either after short-term dosing with a bronchodilator or after several weeks of treatment with an anti-inflammatory medication such as an inhaled steroid. If the patient is doing well, however, pulmonary function tests may be normal. In this case, we can have patients inhale a chemical irritant to stimulate constriction of the airways, leading to a drop in airflow rates. Sometimes we will have patients use a portable, handheld device, called a *peak expiratory flow meter*, to document variability in peak flow rates over time. Health care providers may also use a questionnaire called the *Asthma Control Test* (*ACT*) to quantify how well a patient's symptoms are under control.

Treatment

The goal of asthma treatment is to control symptoms and prevent exacerbations. We classify asthma severity based on frequency of daytime and nocturnal symptoms, number of exacerbations requiring treatment with oral steroids in the past year, and lung function. Most patients will need an inhaled corticosteroid. For those with more symptoms, we can add a long-acting bronchodilator. We have two types of bronchodilators available, one that acts on beta receptors, where stimulation dilates the airways (beta agonists), and one that acts on muscarinic (also called cholinergic) receptors, where blockade dilates the airways. Both types of bronchodilators come in short- and long-acting forms. The short-acting forms we typically reserve as "rescue" inhalers to be used on an as-needed basis. The long-acting forms we view as "maintenance therapy" to help maintain airway patency throughout the entire day. Other "add-on" therapies may include antihistamines and leukotriene antagonists, both oral medications that can help block allergic inflammation. In some patients with mild to moderate asthma with demonstrated allergies to grass pollens or dust mites, immunotherapy ("allergy shots") or sublingual immunotherapy may be considered, although these treatment courses are typically prolonged, and studies suggest only modest benefit.

Patients with severe asthma represent a unique subgroup of patients. In the past few years, we have seen several "biologic" therapies approved for asthma. Biologic therapies are treatments made from living organisms. Most biologic therapies are antibodies that attach either to receptors on cells or to specific inflammatory proteins to block their activity. They are typically delivered through a subcutaneous injection. Many of these newer biologic therapies in asthma still target allergic inflammation, but can help reduce the need for oral steroids. Some patients experience dramatic improvements in symptoms and frequency of exacerbations with the addition of biologic therapy.

Finally, bronchial thermoplasty may be considered, which involves treating the airways in different parts of the lung with radiofrequency energy. The procedure is approved in both the United States and Europe for adults whose severe asthma is not well controlled by inhaled medications, but the trials excluded some of the sickest patients, and long-term benefits appear to be modest.

COPD

Chronic obstructive pulmonary disease (COPD) is a common condition, but it is also a source of confusion for many. The third leading cause of death in the world, COPD is caused by exposure to noxious particles or gases that cause inflammation of the bronchioles and destruction of the alveoli. Bronchiolar inflammation may cause chronic bronchitis, resulting in excess mucus that causes a productive cough. Alveolar destruction causes emphysema. Both of these conditions fall under the COPD umbrella. Although tobacco smoke clearly contributes to the development of COPD, roughly 25 percent of those with COPD have *no personal smoking history*. Certainly, exposure to passive, or secondhand, tobacco smoke plays a role, but other exposures that contribute to COPD include occupational exposures to dusts, gases, and fumes. Relying on biomass fuels (nonfossil, carbon-based energy sources such as wood and solid waste) for cooking and heating in conjunction with poor ventilation is also believed to cause COPD, particularly among women. Three billion people rely on burning biomass and other solid fuels for cooking and heating within their homes. In the United States, it has been estimated that solid fuel is a primary heating source for over 2.5 million households, particularly in rural and low-income areas.[1]

Genetic makeup also contributes to how susceptible an individual is to developing COPD. While a host of genes have been identified that play at least some role, the best-known gene linked to COPD is the gene that encodes for the protein alpha-1 antitrypsin. Alpha-1 antitrypsin is a protein made in the liver that breaks down elastase, a product of neutrophils, a type of white blood cell. Elastase helps to destroy bacteria, but if left unchecked, as with the genetic disorder alpha-1 antitrypsin deficiency, the lung structure can be damaged, leading to emphysema.

Clinical Presentation and Diagnosis

Early in the course of disease, some patients may have no symptoms. Others may have a productive cough. Still others may begin to experience mild shortness of breath, particularly with exertion. However, many research studies now show us that significant CT abnormalities are present in many patients before spirometry results become abnormal. As the airways become more inflamed and the process of lung destruction begins, the lungs begin to trap air at the end of exhalation. Air trapping is due to increased resistance to airflow in the small airways, but also due to a loss of lung elastic recoil. As the lungs become more damaged, oxygen levels may drop and carbon dioxide levels may rise. As with asthma, patients with COPD tend to experience periodic flare-ups, or exacerbations, of their disease, necessitating treatment with antibiotics and steroids.

Patients are diagnosed with COPD based on a consistent history along with spirometry showing "fixed" airflow obstruction, as opposed to the "variable" obstruction we see more commonly in asthma. Fixed obstruction means that no matter when the spirometry is done (a good day or a bad day) and no matter how much medication we might give to open up the airways, some degree of obstruction remains on spirometry. More extensive pulmonary function testing often shows that the lungs are hyperinflated and air cannot be well expelled at the end of exhalation. Unfortunately, only a third of patients in the United States who are given a diagnosis of COPD have had any kind of pulmonary function testing at all.[2] This leads to both misdiagnosis and underdiagnosis. Some estimates suggest as many as half of the patients with COPD in the United States have not yet been given a diagnosis.

As with asthma, symptoms may be further assessed with a simple questionnaire such as the COPD Assessment Test (CAT), which is a short questionnaire that helps us to quantify how symptomatic a patient is. While CT imaging is not currently considered "standard of care" for COPD, there are many reasons why patients with COPD may undergo imaging. This includes screening for lung cancer or to be evaluated for advanced therapies.

Treatment

For individuals who are smoking, it's never too late to stop. This is the best treatment we have for tobacco-associated COPD. If there is a factor in one's home or work environment that contributes to poor air quality, remedying that is also important. Examples include wearing a respirator at a dusty job or avoiding secondhand smoke. With respect to medicines, the mainstay of treatment for many years has been inhaled bronchodilators. Bronchodilators can improve lung function and relieve symptoms. Inhaled corticosteroids can also help improve lung function and symptoms, but are likely most helpful in reducing exacerbations, particularly among individuals with higher blood eosinophil counts (a type of white blood cell). Studies also suggest that among patients who have frequent exacerbations, being on two types of bronchodilators in addition to inhaled corticosteroids ("triple therapy") may improve survival.

As for patients with alpha-1 antitrypsin deficiency, we can supplement this enzyme through injections, which may help to preserve lung function. Supplemental oxygen has been shown to improve survival in patients who have low levels of oxygen all the time (pulse oximetry under 88 percent). For patients who have milder impairments and whose oxygen saturation drops only occasionally, such as with activity, there is not strong evidence that oxygen improves clinical outcomes,[3] although it is still widely prescribed in this setting. One of the best nonpharmacological treatments we have for COPD is pulmonary rehabilitation, a comprehensive, medically supervised exercise and education program that can improve symptoms and exercise capacity.

Several more invasive treatments are also available. Lung volume reduction surgery (LVRS) benefits patients with emphysema predominantly in the upper portions of the lungs. In this procedure, the upper portions of the lungs are surgically removed, thereby improving the mechanics of breathing. This moves the diaphragm closer to its normal resting position. Recently, one-way valves that can deflate emphysematous portions of the lung have also been approved for use in the United States and Europe. This procedure also improves breathing mechanics, making patients less short of breath and able to exercise more. This procedure does not require surgery and can be performed using a bronchoscope. In the most advanced cases of COPD, lung transplant may be the only option.

Cystic Fibrosis

Cystic fibrosis (CF) is a genetic disorder affecting roughly 70,000 people worldwide, more common among whites and less common among Blacks and Asians. While CF is thought of as a lung disease, it causes multiple problems beyond the lungs, affecting the pancreas, gastrointestinal tract, skin, and male reproductive organs. There are reports of CF dating back to 1650, when high sweat salinity in children was associated with premature death. In fact, an old Irish proverb stated, "If your baby tastes of salt, he is not long for this world." The noted association of very salty sweat led to the modern hypothesis that abnormal chloride channels may be central to the disease. Sweat chloride testing remains a key diagnostic test for cystic fibrosis.

The first comprehensive report describing the clinical features of CF was published in 1938. By 1946, scientists examining inheritance patterns deduced that CF was caused by a recessive mutation (genetic disease that manifests when two bad copies of a gene are present). The gene responsible for CF was finally localized to chromosome 7 in the 1980s and its exact location pinpointed in 1989.

We now know that the *CFTR* (cystic fibrosis transmembrane conductance regulator) gene contains the code for a protein that serves as a cell membrane channel, transporting chloride ions out of cells lining the respiratory tract. Multiple different types of mutations within this gene have been described, but they all lead to a lack or malfunction of this critical protein.

Clinical Presentation and Diagnosis

Decreased chloride and bicarbonate secretion create thick lung secretions, resulting in abnormal mucociliary clearance. Patients with CF may also have impaired flow of bile and pancreatic digestive enzymes, which can lead to liver disease, malnutrition, and bowel blockages. The biggest lung problem patients with CF have is chronic lung infections. Thick secretions cause the ciliary escalator in the lungs to fail. Hence, this built-in defense system can no longer adequately clear bacteria. Bacteria begin to establish residence in the airways of CF patients at an early age. One type of bacteria in particular, *Pseudomonas aeruginosa*, actually creates biofilms, organized bacterial communities that can coat the airways, making them particularly difficult to eradicate. The lungs develop not only airflow obstruction as measured on pulmonary function testing, but a thickening and dilation of the airways we call bronchiectasis. Bronchiectasis can be seen in other lung conditions, but is a prominent feature of patients with CF. Similar to other obstructive lung diseases like asthma and COPD, patients with CF also experience flare-ups, or exacerbations, of their lung disease.

Many countries, including the United States, Western European nations, and Australia, have implemented newborn screening programs for CF, which measure a compound in the blood called *immunoreactive trypsinogen*, a marker of pancreatic injury. If trypsinogen is abnormally elevated, further evaluation is recommended, including evaluation for sinus, lung, and gastrointestinal abnormalities and measurement of sweat chloride concentration from the skin. If this testing is equivocal, genetic testing for common, known *CFTR* mutations is typically performed to confirm or rule out the diagnosis of CF. If adults present with clinical features suspicious for CF, sweat chloride testing is also the first test usually performed. However, as new therapies that target specific mutations are now available, genotyping really should be obtained in all patients to understand who is eligible for these specialized treatments.

Treatment

The Cystic Fibrosis Foundation funds over 130 care centers to provide comprehensive disease management. Treatment for CF through one of these centers is highly recommended if possible, as it provides patients with access to the most up-to-date, standardized, and comprehensive care. As with other airway-centered conditions, bronchodilators are often used in CF. Patients with CF who have asthmatic features to their disease (airway hyperreactivity) may also benefit from inhaled corticosteroids.

Other treatments are more specific to CF. This includes nebulized solutions that patients breathe in as a mist, such as hypertonic saline to help break mucus and restore ciliary escalator function. Another drug called dornase alfa (Pulmozyme) breaks up DNA in lung secretions to reduce their viscosity, making them less sticky. Inhaled antibiotics are also frequently used. Improving mechanical clearance of secretions is also an important part of CF treatment that may include physical percussion and vibration of the chest, percussion vests, and other devices that cause mechanical vibration of the lungs to loosen secretions. These types of mechanical clearance techniques can also be helpful for other patients with bronchiectasis that we see in lung conditions outside of CF. Regular exercise can also help to loosen and clear secretions. Inhaled antibiotics and oral antibiotics may also be used.

One of the most exciting advances in pulmonary medicine has been the development of CF transmembrane conductance regulator (CFTR) modulators. These drugs uniquely target specific defects in the CFTR protein to restore function to the protein. For patients with specific *CFTR* mutations, these revolutionary therapies are anticipated to profoundly improve quality of life and longevity. The goal now is to get as many eligible patients as possible started on these medications early in the course of their disease and to continue developing treatments for those not helped with the currently approved drugs.

Interstitial Lung Diseases

Interstitial lung disease (ILD), which is also called *diffuse parenchymal lung disease*, represents a host of scarring disorders of the lung (fibrosis) from multiple known and unknown causes. ILDs also represent some of the biggest diagnostic and therapeutic challenges for pulmonary clinicians. Some of these disorders have characteristic scarring patterns; the scarring in others, when severe enough, can look the same no matter what the cause.

For some ILDs, we understand what causes them. For instance, autoimmune diseases such as rheumatoid arthritis and lupus can cause lung inflammation. Other interstitial lung diseases are caused by occupational or environmental exposures, including asbestos and silica, or antigen inhalation, as is the case with hypersensitivity pneumonitis. Both chemotherapy and radiation therapy used in the treatment of cancers may cause fibrosis of the lung. Other medications, such as methotrexate (used to treat rheumatological diseases) and amiodarone (used to treat cardiac arrhythmias), can cause inflammatory conditions in the lung.

For other ILDs, we don't understand what causes them. This includes idiopathic pulmonary fibrosis (IPF) and nonspecific interstitial pneumonia (NSIP), both of which have a characteristic appearance under the microscope. NSIP may have no identifiable cause or in some cases is associated with connective tissue diseases. This group also includes diseases that present more acutely or subacutely, including cryptogenic organizing pneumonia, which may look like pneumonia in multiple parts of the lung but without evidence of infection, and acute interstitial pneumonia, which can rapidly lead to respiratory failure. While most people think of smoking as the cause of COPD, it can also cause other lung diseases, including respiratory bronchiolitis interstitial lung disease (RBILD), and desquamative interstitial pneumonia (DIP).

Other disorders in this category include sarcoidosis, which causes tiny nodules in the lungs that may go away but in other cases cause scarring in the lungs. Lymphangioleiomyomatosis (LAM) and pulmonary Langerhans cell histiocytosis (PLCH) are also included in this group, as are eosinophilic lung diseases, in which white blood cells called eosinophils accumulate in the lung, and pulmonary alveolar proteinosis (PAP), in which excess surfactant builds up in the lung.

Clinical Presentation and Diagnosis

Symptoms differ, depending on the specific disease, but many of these diseases are slowly progressive and tend to get picked up only late in the disease course. Shortness of breath is a common symptom of many ILDs. Patients with IPF may develop an intractable dry cough. A few ILDs have more unique presentations. For instance, in addition to affecting the lungs, sarcoidosis can impact almost every organ system of the body. Sarcoidosis is often identified incidentally on a chest X-ray when enlarged lymph nodes are seen at the center of the lung, just as the bronchi branch out (called the "hilum"). It also commonly presents with cough, shortness of breath, fatigue, and weight loss. LAM, a rare lung disease only affecting women, may present with a pneumothorax.

Beyond the clinical history, imaging is one of the most important tools we have to diagnose interstitial lung diseases.

Both the type and location of abnormalities can help in diagnosis. Early in the course of interstitial lung disease we may see a radiological abnormality termed "ground glass opacification." This refers to an abnormality seen on the CT scan that partially but not completely obscures the underlying lung structure. Sometimes ground glass opacities resolve with treatment, meaning they represent inflammation. In other cases, such abnormalities represent lung scarring. The connective tissue that binds the lung together may also be impacted by scarring. Radiologists sometimes call this a "reticular pattern." In end-stage lung disease, we can see a CT pattern called "honeycombing." This is where having pulmonologists working with radiologists in ILD case conferences can be especially helpful. We may try to obtain biopsies via bronchoscopy. Sometimes these small bronchoscopy biopsies are enough for diagnosis, but it is not uncommon for patients to ultimately need a more invasive surgical lung biopsy to make a diagnosis.

Treatment

For interstitial lung diseases associated with a specific cause, treating the underlying cause can benefit the lung. For lung disease associated with rheumatologic diseases, this usually involves a combination of steroids and/or immunosuppressants. For drug- or exposure-induced ILD, removing the offending agent is the most important intervention. For years, our general approach to most ILDs has been a combination of steroids and other immunosuppressive agents. However, in 2014, two drugs—nintedanib and pirfenidone—were approved for idiopathic pulmonary fibrosis. Since then, nintedanib has also been approved for treatment of scleroderma-related ILD and more broadly for multiple types of progressive fibrosing interstitial lung diseases, including NSIP, chronic hypersensitivity pneumonitis, and autoimmune ILD.

A few interstitial lung diseases have unique treatments. This includes LAM, for which a class of immunosuppressive drugs, the mTOR inhibitors, act on the genetic mutation on the *TSC* gene responsible for the disease. For pulmonary alveolar proteinosis, the initial treatment is to drown the lungs in saline. Under anesthesia, we use a special double lumen endotracheal tube that ventilates each lung separately. We then sequentially flood each lung with normal saline and then suck back up as much fluid as we can. This helps to wash out the surfactant that has built up. Administration of a protein called GM-CSF may also have efficacy in PAP. For all ILDs, treatment requires close monitoring and fine-tuning.

Lung Cancer

Lung cancer causes the most cancer-related deaths in the Western world. Roughly 10 percent of long-term smokers will eventually be diagnosed with lung cancer. Fortunately, in recent years, prevalence of smoking among adults is on the decline, although 10 to 15 percent of those with lung cancer never smoked. Among the nonsmokers who develop cancer, women appear to be at significantly greater risk than men.[4] Looked at another way, in the United States, roughly 20 percent of lung cancer in women occurs in those who have never smoked.[5] Among these non-smokers, passive smoke exposure is a likely factor. Air pollution, radon exposure, and perhaps genetics may also play a role. Other lung conditions associated with inflammation also appear to be associated with increased risk for lung cancer. These include pulmonary fibrosis and emphysema. It is notable that whereas lung cancer incidence (new case rate) and mortality (death rate) are similar between Black and white women in the United States, they are significantly higher for Black men as compared to white men.

Lung cancer can be broken into multiple types based on the cell type they originally derive from. Adenocarcinoma is the most common type of lung cancer, representing roughly 40 percent of lung cancers in the United States. Adenocarcinoma arises from mucus-producing glandular cells residing in the lung airways. Squamous cell carcinoma is the second most common subtype, accounting for roughly 20 percent of lung cancers in the United States. It arises from epithelial cells in the more central portion of the tracheobronchial tree. Small cell lung cancer causes approximately 15 percent of lung cancers in the United States and has the strongest association to smoking. Large cell carcinoma lacks some of the identifiable features of adenocarcinoma and squamous cell carcinoma and currently represents 3 percent of US lung cancers. Carcinoid tumors account for 1 to 2 percent of US lung cancers and are the most frequent tumor of the lung in children. These cancers are typically benign and not associated with tobacco use.

Clinical Presentation and Diagnosis

Most patients with lung cancer initially have no symptoms, leading to diagnosis at later stages. Sometimes tumors are picked up earlier as an incidental finding on chest imaging. When patients do present with symptoms, they may report cough, shortness of breath, coughing up blood, or weight loss. In fact, in one study where patients were screened to detect lung cancers in a high-risk population, 40 percent had symptoms. However, of the patients generally diagnosed with cancer, roughly 75 percent have symptoms, emphasizing the point that lung cancer tends to be discovered late. However, we now have data from several large lung cancer screening studies suggesting that screening for lung cancer among high-risk patient populations can reduce deaths. Chest CT is much more sensitive than standard chest X-rays for detecting lung cancers. The National Lung Screening Trial (NLST) was the first large, randomized trial to demonstrate reduced risk for death with lung cancer screening. In the United States, Medicare Part B now covers a low radiation dose screening chest CT on an annual basis for those between the ages of 55 and 77 who do not currently have symptoms of lung cancer, are a current or former smoker within the past 15 years, have smoked on average a pack a day for 30 years, and have an order from a doctor. However, in March of 2020, new guidance from the US Preventive Services Task Force has recommended expanding screening to individuals aged 50 to 80 with a 20 pack-year smoking history. As of April 2021, the Centers for Medicare and Medicaid Services (CMS) has not updated their national coverage determination to reflect the new guidelines.

CT imaging is usually the first step to identifying and characterizing lung cancers. Part of lung cancer evaluation is not only confirming the existence of cancer and its type, but also assessing the extent of its spread. We call this "staging." Here we are looking to determine what parts of the lung are involved, but also what lymph nodes within the thoracic cavity might also have cancer that has spread. We may sometimes see fluid around the involved lung and must determine whether cancer cells are present in this fluid, which informs the extent of spread. Often a PET scan may be ordered to help stage the lung cancer. PET scans are typically done on the entire body so that "hot spots" outside the lung can also be identified. Because of frequent spread to the brain, imaging of the brain with either MRI or CT is also often included in the workup of small cell lung cancers, particularly if it is known that the cancer has spread to lymph nodes. Once the areas of concern are identified, the next step is to obtain a tissue biopsy, which may be performed with the use of bronchoscopy or a CT-guided needle. If there is concern for spread, we try to biopsy the area that would yield the highest disease stage for the purposes of treatment planning.

Treatment

The treatment of lung cancer has evolved significantly over the past few years, in part due to the discovery of molecular biomarkers that can help to guide therapies. We still broadly categorize lung cancers into non-small cell lung cancer (adenocarcinoma, squamous cell carcinoma) and small cell lung cancer. Lower-stage non-small cell cancers can generally be removed surgically. These patients with lower-stage cancers may or may not be candidates for chemotherapy. If patients are not well enough to undergo surgery, radiation therapy can be curative in some cases. Curative treatments for middle-stage cancers usually include chemotherapy. For patients with more advanced non-small cell cancers, palliative chemotherapy or radiation therapy can be very effective, though not curative, in most cases. As with all cancers, such cases are typically discussed at a multidisciplinary hospital tumor board to identify the best treatment plan for each patient. For small cell lung cancers, if the cancer is limited to half the chest (right or left), radiation therapy is typically the initial treatment option. For more extensive disease, chemotherapy is the primary treatment of choice. Small cell cancer can be cured in roughly 20 to 25 percent of patients with limited disease. For more extensive disease, while chemotherapy is life prolonging, a cure typically cannot be achieved.

Some of the biggest advances in lung cancer therapy in the past 20 years have come from the ability to genotype mutations in cancer cells to personalize chemotherapy regimens for individual patients. As we have become more sophisticated in our understanding of how tumor cells operate, several key alterations in cell cycle or growth regulation pathways have been identified that drive rapid growth. Highly targeted chemotherapies can now target very specific mutations. Patients with advanced stage non-small cell lung cancers should ideally have their tumors assessed for the presence of specific mutations. Certain chemotherapy agents have been identified that appear to be more effective when specific types of mutations are present. If no such mutations are identified, patients may still be candidates for a newer class of cancer drugs called *immune checkpoint inhibitors* that boost the ability of the body's immune system to fight cancer.

Pulmonary Circulatory Disorders

Disorders of the pulmonary circulation typically involve the blood vessels running from the right side of the heart, through the lung, and back into the left side of the heart. The most common disorders include blood clots that lodge in the lung, called *pulmonary emboli*. It is estimated that acute pulmonary emboli account for over 200,000 hospital admissions in the United States annually. Acute pulmonary emboli can be fatal, with up to 10 percent of patients dying from the condition. These clots most commonly originate from the deep veins in the upper legs but can also come from the pelvis and upper extremities.

A variety of disorders, including clots, can cause blood pressure in the pulmonary vascular system to be elevated. We call this pulmonary hypertension. Pulmonary hypertension is further broken down into five groups. Group 1 is caused by abnormalities within the pulmonary arteries themselves. Pulmonary arterial hypertension (PAH) can be due to inherited genetic mutations, develop in association with connective tissue diseases such as scleroderma, or have no known cause (idiopathic). Group 2 is due to failure of the left side of the heart to adequately push blood forward, causing a backup of blood into the lungs with a subsequent increase in the pressures within the pulmonary arteries. This is the most common form of pulmonary hypertension. Group 3 is due to chronic lung diseases (such as COPD), where lung destruction and/or low oxygen levels cause vascular damage. Group 4 is due to chronic pulmonary emboli. Group 5 patients do not clearly fit into any of the previous groups and include patients with blood disorders such as sickle cell disease and other systemic or metabolic disorders.

Clinical Presentation and Diagnosis

Patients with acute pulmonary emboli typically present with acute shortness of breath followed by chest pain. However, patients may range from having no symptoms to presenting with shock or sudden death. The onset of pulmonary hypertension is usually more insidious, as it takes time to develop. The symptoms may also be more nonspecific, including shortness of breath with exertion and fatigue. Chronic pulmonary hypertension can ultimately lead to right heart failure with subsequent accumulation of fluid in the abdomen and legs.

Diagnosis of pulmonary emboli depends first on a good clinical history. Patients who have been immobile or have malignancy are at particularly high risk for developing clots. Clinicians typically combine their clinical suspicion along with a test for blood D-dimer (a protein fragment that comes from blood clots) to guide further testing. CT pulmonary angiogram is currently the diagnostic modality of choice. However, in certain circumstances, such as when contrast dye is contraindicated, a V/Q scan may be used.

The workup of pulmonary hypertension typically begins with an echocardiogram, which helps assess the function of both sides of the heart. Pressure in the pulmonary arteries can be estimated based on the rate of blood backflow through the tricuspid valve (where venous blood returning from the body enters the right side of the heart). Depending on the level of clinical suspicion and the echocardiogram results, some patients will go on to a right heart catheterization. In this procedure, a catheter is threaded into the right side of the heart into the pulmonary arteries so that the pressure can be accurately measured. If pulmonary hypertension is diagnosed, then further diagnostic testing is conducted to identify possible causes.

Treatment

The treatment for pulmonary emboli involves anticoagulation. The specific treatment depends on the clinical situation but may include IV heparin, a subcutaneous injectable form of heparin, pills that inhibit specific parts of the clotting cascade (thrombin inhibitors and factor Xa inhibitors), or warfarin. In severe cases, we may administer medication to break up the clot (thrombolytic medication) or try to directly remove the clot. In other cases, where anticoagulation is not possible, a filter may be placed in the inferior vena cava to prevent further clots from entering the lungs. Treatment for pulmonary hypertension depends on the type. However, we only have specific therapies for Group 1.

Respiratory Failure

When the lungs of patients with chronic lung conditions can no longer support them, transplant may be the only option. The first lung transplant was attempted in 1963, but it wasn't for another 20 years that the procedure was ultimately successful. Unfortunately, long-term survival is still only around 50 percent at five years. The lung is one of the few transplanted organs that is still exposed daily to environmental and infectious insults, making protection of the transplanted lung challenging. However, for some patients this is our only option. Patients require a complex regimen of immunosuppressive medications to prevent organ rejection and prophylactic antibiotics to prevent infection. Lung transplant evaluation is a complex process that typically takes months. Due to a limited donor pool, some patients may wait years to receive a lung transplant or, unfortunately, not live long enough to obtain one. While long-term outcomes vary widely between patients, I have several patients who received transplants over 15 years ago and are still doing quite well.

If respiratory failure is temporary, brought on, for instance, by severe pneumonia, we have several treatment options. But first we must remember the lung's two main jobs: to get oxygen in and carbon dioxide out. So we must identify which piece of this is failing in order to establish the best supportive device for an individual patient. Most simple is supplemental oxygen delivered to the nose via a loose-fitting nasal cannula or mask. When even more oxygen is needed, another mode of oxygen delivery called *high-flow nasal cannula* (*HFNC*) may be used. In HFNC, heated, humidified air increases the water content in the mucus lining the airways, which can help get rid of secretions and decrease the work of breathing. The high-flow rates combined with a special, tight-fitting nasal cannula drives air in and allows higher, more accurate delivery of oxygen. We also have ways of forcing air into the lungs using "noninvasive" equipment that involves a mask being strapped to a patient's face and air being blown into the lungs. This is referred to as *noninvasive ventilation (NIV)*. In acute respiratory failure, NIV is typically delivered with a mask interface attached to a mechanical ventilator using a mode called *BiPAP (bilevel positive airway pressure)*, which provides pressure at two settings during both inspiration and expiration. BiPAP can improve oxygenation and also help get rid of excess carbon dioxide. Not all patients may be candidates for NIV due to the level of their alertness and severity of their condition.

Finally, we have *invasive mechanical ventilation*. If you've ever undergone a major operation, then you were most likely supported by a mechanical ventilator during the procedure. Mechanical ventilation involves an endotracheal tube that is introduced through the mouth and extends past the vocal cords and into the trachea. This tube is then connected to a mechanical ventilator and allows physicians the highest degree of control. Here we can increase oxygen either by turning up the level of oxygen delivered or by continuing to deliver some pressure into the lungs at the end of the breath. This is known as *PEEP*, or *positive end expiratory pressure*. We can get rid of carbon dioxide by either speeding up the respiratory rate or making the volume of air delivered with each breath larger.

Several other things about mechanical ventilation are important to know. The first is that we normally breathe by negative pressure, not positive pressure. Hence, mechanical ventilation is inherently uncomfortable for patients. The ventilator can be placed into a mode that senses when the patient wants to take a breath and assists at the appropriate time. However, in reality it is still uncomfortable, and patients may require heavy sedation. The second thing to realize is that both too much oxygen and breaths that are too large can injure the lungs. Hence, doctors are always balancing treating the acute problem while not creating a new one. In some cases, the lung injury is so bad that we initiate something called *ECMO*, which stands for *extracorporeal membranous oxygen*. This involves placing very large catheters into the central veins, drawing blood out, and running it through a machine that oxygenates the blood and delivers it back to the body. This is a very complicated, labor-intensive procedure that is typically available only at large medical centers.

Stem Cell Therapy

In recent years, we have unfortunately seen aggressive direct-to-patient marketing by some medical centers touting the benefits of stem cell therapies for end-stage lung disease. While the potential of stem cells to treat both lung and non-lung diseases is being studied, no such treatments have yet proved effective in rigorously performed clinical trials for patients with lung diseases. Many patient and physician organizations have come out with official statements warning how little is known about these proposed therapies. The FDA has begun increased enforcement of regulations and oversight of stem cell clinics. All such therapies for the lung at this time should be considered experimental and only conducted within the auspices of a regulated clinical trial with appropriate oversight and outcome assessment. All credible trials are registered on the National Library of Medicine Clinical Trials website.

Chapter 6

The Fifth Vital Sign

The COVID-19 pandemic has strained the global health care system, in some places to the breaking point. It has also raised the profile of lung disease as well as lung health. The importance of understanding how to protect and preserve lung function has never been fully appreciated until this moment. While massive efforts have been undertaken to develop vaccines and effective treatments, health care providers have relied heavily on an existing knowledge base of how the lungs work, fight infection, and recover from severe attack. Yet we now realize that it is not enough. As of early 2021, nearly 3 million individuals have died from COVID-19, the majority from respiratory failure. The pandemic has also revealed that much of the lay public lacks even a basic understanding of how the lungs work or how we might protect our lungs. Even before the pandemic, the lungs have been a relatively low priority target for both research funding and public education. But now we have arrived at a moment of reckoning. We now understand that safeguarding lung health is crucial to our overall health and survival. This leads us to two questions. The first, How did we get here?, is followed closely by the second, Where do we go from here?

A Brief History Lesson

Much of our basic understanding of human health comes from "bench" research done in laboratories and from clinical trials involving human beings. Such research can have a profound impact on improving human health. For example, medical research has fueled an abundance of treatments for high blood pressure and high cholesterol. Overall deaths from cardiovascular disease have plummeted since the late 1960s, a testament to the success of medical research and historically robust funding for cardiovascular diseases.

During this same time period, however, overall deaths from chronic lung disease have been relatively flat. Even more concerning for doctors and patients alike, the number of new treatments for the most common lung conditions remains small as compared to other common chronic health conditions. Funding for lung research has long held a position of lower priority. Consider the heart and the lungs. They both sit encased within the chest. Conceptually, our study of these two organs could have evolved similarly, but they didn't. At key points in history, their paths diverged.

John Hutchinson's work to develop the spirometer in the 1840s was hugely important, but the device was not widely accepted.[1] To this day, measurement of lung function remains an obscure practice to most of the general public. Contrast this to the sphygmomanometer, the device commonly used to measure blood pressure. Blood pressure cuffs are present in nearly every patient exam room in the world and familiar to almost everyone. Blood pressure is considered one of the four "vital signs" in addition to temperature, heart rate, and respiratory rate. Yet, the predecessor of the modern-day sphygmomanometer was introduced roughly 50 years *after* the spirometer, by Italian physician Scipione Riva-Rocci in 1896.

It appears that blood pressure measurement was especially embraced by physicians at the beginning of the twentieth century, when Russian physician Nikolai Korotkoff expanded the utility of the blood pressure cuff by combining its use with a stethoscope. The combination of tools allows measurement of both systolic and diastolic blood pressure. Medical historians posit that at the time, it was important for physicians to distinguish their skill set from that of nurses and technical assistants. The addition of the stethoscope made the measurement of blood pressure a procedure worthy of a physician's skill level.

Yet the value of blood pressure measurement wasn't established until well *after* its widespread adoption. We now know that blood pressure helps predict the risk for heart attacks and strokes. Given our heavy dependence on data in the era of modern medicine, instruments must now prove their value by providing unique diagnostic or prognostic information before they are widely accepted. However, in the early 1900s, physician sentiment played a much larger role in the implementation of new techniques.

While blood pressure measurements were taking off, advancements in pulmonary function testing lagged until lung health issues related to commercial manufacturing and widespread use of cigarettes increased the recognition of lung disease. But even now, when easy-to-use digital spirometers are widely available, many primary care offices do not own a single machine. The reasons for this are numerous, but it has been suggested that we chest physicians share some of the blame for shrouding spirometry in mystery and overcomplicating the procedure.

For instance, we require patients to repeat pulmonary function tests several times to ensure that the measures are reproducible. Reported values are highly accurate. The pulmonologist Thomas Petty lamented the underutilization of spirometry in medicine by quoting a famous Pogo comic strip line: "We have met the enemy . . . and he is us!"[2] Routine blood pressure measurements done in a physician's office are typically not performed with the same level of rigor. For precise blood pressure measurements, 5 minutes of rest would be enforced and the blood pressure reading would be an average of multiple measurements. We pulmonologists have held spirometry to a higher standard. This requirement for perfection has arguably contributed to decreased widespread use.

Ironically, spirometry is now in a bit of a no-win situation. The US National Preventive Services Task Force recommends against widespread population screening with spirometry, as the evidence base that it would alter clinical outcomes has yet to be established. Yet, as most lung disease in the United States is picked up relatively late in the course of disease, the majority of clinical trials for diseases like COPD have had difficulty demonstrating that medications can alter the course of the disease. This is rather like evaluating erosion prevention measures on a plot of land where much soil has already been lost. No matter what you do at this point, the soil is already gone. It will be difficult to establish the evidence base to support wider use of spirometry unless we identify patients with earlier disease. And so the cycle continues.

Imagine a scenario where half of the patients with hypertension are never told they have high blood pressure at all. Of those who are told they have hypertension, only a third of those individuals ever get their blood pressure measured. Medications may be initiated or even changed around, but again the blood pressure isn't assessed. This pretty much sums up the state of spirometry for COPD in the United States.

What does this mean for patients? In my own practice at the University of Michigan, I run a clinic where we see patients with COPD after they have been in the hospital for an exacerbation. In our experience, roughly 10 to 15 percent don't even have COPD when we bring them into the office for testing. At the other end of the spectrum, I have had patients referred to me for initial consultation with significantly advanced stages of disease. One such individual had been shrugging off his symptoms of shortness of breath for a while. By the time he made it to my office, his lung function was so impaired that I had to begin discussions with him about lung transplant on his very first visit. For other patients, we have discovered completely unrelated lung conditions, such as pulmonary fibrosis, heart failure, asthma, and even a paralyzed diaphragm, as alternative explanations for the hospitalization.

So how exactly did blood pressure develop the massive evidence base that currently supports its measurement? In 1932, Franklin Delano Roosevelt was running for the highest office in the land, and his campaign released his health records, including a blood pressure measurement of 140/100 mm Hg.[3] Normal blood pressure is currently defined as under 120/80 mm Hg. Today, Roosevelt's measurements would have raised alarm. But at the time, no one blinked. In fact, understanding of cardiovascular disease at that time was so poor that when FDR was elected 32nd president of the United States, he chose an ear, nose, and throat specialist to be his personal physician during the presidency. Over the next few years, his blood pressure continued to rise, recorded at 188/105 mm Hg in 1941. By 1944, he was diagnosed with heart failure, and in 1945, President Roosevelt died from a stroke. His blood pressure around that time was 300/190 mm Hg. Today we know that had his blood pressure been treated, he may have avoided both heart failure and stroke.

Our understanding of blood pressure and its relationship to cardiovascular disease at that time was quite limited. But following President Roosevelt's death, in 1947 legislators drafted the National Heart Act, providing funding for one of the most important epidemiological studies ever conducted, the Framingham Heart Study (FHS). Framingham was the first long-term study of its kind. The goal was to use the citizens of Framingham, Massachusetts, to understand factors that predispose to the development of cardiovascular disease. The city of Framingham was chosen in part because it was near Harvard Medical School and in part due to the enthusiastic response from the community itself. Over the subsequent 70 years, the FHS has shaped our understanding of hypertension, obesity, and cholesterol as contributors to cardiovascular disease. It has provided the evidence basis for a slew of treatments we now have to both prevent and treat cardiovascular disease. Maintaining continuous funding for a study of this scale that would focus on not only the original participants but also their descendants has proved to be a feat in itself. The success of this study is a testament to the dedication of the many researchers that have overseen it and to the community involved. The study would ultimately need not only NIH funding but also private and corporate support at points in its history. Yet over time, mortality from cardiovascular disease has steadily declined, and the nation has been able to turn its attention to heart disease prevention as opposed to disease treatment alone. It is due in part to the FHS that we even speak about the concept of heart health and understand how risk factors such as blood pressure and cholesterol can be modified to maintain health and prevent disease.

Fueled by these early successes, cardiovascular disease research funding remains relatively robust. Data from 2019 released by the World Health Organization (WHO) indicate that as a disease category, cardiovascular disease comes in with the fifth highest number of research grants.[4] It is true that ischemic heart disease and stroke are the number one and two causes of death worldwide and clearly worthy of further study. However, COPD and lower respiratory infections are the third and fourth leading causes of death globally. Yet in terms of research grant numbers, WHO reports that respiratory diseases and respiratory infections come in thirteenth and seventeenth, respectively.

According to the same WHO report, the NIH represents one of the largest sources of grants for medical research in the world, outside the private sector. Physicians and medical scientists, especially within the United States, rely heavily on NIH funding to support their work. As an organization, the NIH funds an incredible amount of research spanning almost every aspect of human health. Further analyses of NIH spending demonstrate that historically there has been a largely predictable relationship between the amount of disability a disease causes, measured in something called *disability-adjusted life years* (a quantification of life lost due to living at less than full health), and the amount of money spent.[5] However, there are some outliers. Public perception and patient advocacy are additional factors that influence funding.[6] Diseases that carry stigma as potentially being "self-inflicted" and related to "bad habits" such as smoking or alcoholism have historically fared less well than nonstigmatized diseases. Both lung cancer and COPD, for instance, have received less funding over time than might be expected relative to their overall impact on public health.

As a society, we must remember that health behaviors play a role in many, many diseases beyond the most obvious associations. It is ultimately not helpful to stratify funding and care for patients based on the perceived percentage they may have played in causing their own health problems. Asthma is common in childhood, with greater prevalence among those with

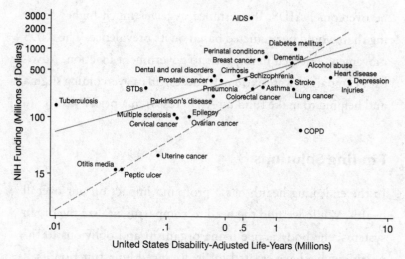

NIH funding (2006) versus disease burden (2004) for 29 common diseases in the United States. Disease burden is measured in disability-adjusted life years (DALY), which is the sum of life years lost due to premature deaths as well as years of healthy life lost due to living with disability. Here, the two lines represent two models used to predict NIH funding for various diseases based on the disease burden they are responsible for, with the difference between the solid and dashed lines being that the model for the dashed line is forced to start at zero (no disease burden equals no funding). The dots represent actual funding. In general, actual versus predicted funding are similar. However, note that funding for both COPD and lung cancer fall below predicted values, with COPD funding having the greatest disparity between actual and predicted of the 29 common diseases examined.

lower socioeconomic status and among non-Hispanic Blacks. COPD tends to afflict older individuals who on average also have lower socioeconomic status and live in more rural areas than their non-COPD counterparts. Both of these groups face challenges simply accessing basic health services, making organizing patient advocacy a herculean task. However, stigma can be overcome. AIDS, for instance, receives much higher funding than would be predicted based on its prevalence. The AIDS movement emerged in response to government inaction. Advocacy campaigns were extremely successful in overcoming stigma and helping to make funding AIDS research a priority.

Finding Solutions

In the end, lung health has a profound impact on our overall health. While we find the need to compartmentalize the organ systems, the body is one living organism and oblivious to the partitions we have created for it. Reduced lung function itself is a predictor not only of overall mortality, but also death from heart disease, reminding us of just how interconnected the parts of our body are. While air pollution impacts the lungs, ultrafine particulate matter is actually absorbed into the bloodstream, where it causes inflammation, contributing not only to heart disease but also to obesity and diabetes.[7] Anxiety and depression are also common among individuals with lung disease. As individuals and members of a global community, understanding these connections is imperative to creating a healthier society.

Knowing this, the question becomes, How can we preserve human lung health? We must first raise awareness. As pulmonologists, we have not done enough to explain the importance of safeguarding lung health over the life span, to the public or even to our colleagues. We must also focus on prevention. Tobacco is arguably the single largest contributor to lung disease and one of the most heavily marketed consumer products in the United States. The advertising spending for the five largest cigarette manufacturers was nearly $9 billion in 2016. While Tobacco 21 legislation passed in 2019 raises the legal age to purchase tobacco from 18 to 21, more protections are needed. The FDA has also been slow to regulate e-cigarettes. Increasing cigarette taxes, curbing marketing (particularly to youth), better enforcement of Tobacco 21 legislation, and extending smoke-free legislation to cover outdoor spaces to discourage smokers and protect bystanders would make a huge difference.

We need to fight harder to protect air quality. Roughly 40 percent of all Americans live with dangerous levels of air pollution. The United States adopted the Clean Air Act in 1970. Total emissions of major air pollutants subsequently dropped by 63 percent from 1980 to 2015, but there are constant threats from those who would seek to make protections weaker. Climate change contributes to increased ozone levels in the air we breathe. Hotter temperatures combined with lack of rainfall have increased particle pollution. What this means is that even greater protections need to be put in place. From a global perspective, air pollution in certain parts of the world, such as India and China, are frequently at dangerous levels. Coordinated efforts to reduce air pollution, such as the C40 Clean Air Cities Declaration, and greenhouse gas emissions, such as the United Nations Paris Agreement, are imperative.

We must also redouble our research efforts toward understanding how lung disease develops and finding new therapies. The UK National Institute for Health Research recently committed 12 percent of its total grant allocation to responsive respiratory research, which has led to the formation of a Global Health Respiratory Network to synergize research programs across the globe. The NIH recently partnered with the American Lung Association to initiate a study enrolling young adults to understand the determinants of lung disease over the life course. There are several other studies around the world that are enrolling large numbers of younger individuals at risk for lung disease, which will in time contribute to our body of knowledge on what shapes human lung health as well as lung disease.

The pharmaceutical industry also plays a key role in developing new medicines for patients. It is most likely that near-term innovations could occur at two ends of the disease spectrum. The first is for the most severely ill patients. Such individuals drive much of our health care costs. Because these patients deteriorate quickly, they are also easier to study. Here we have recently seen the development of a class of drugs called *biologics* that help keep the sickest patients, particularly those with severe asthma, out of the hospital. These drugs differ from chemically synthesized pharmaceuticals in that they are either in whole or in part isolated from living sources, including humans, plants, and microbes. While they are expensive to produce, they are able to target specific biological pathways, which means that the likelihood for clinical success with such drugs is also high. For some patients with severe asthma, these medications have made it possible to discontinue or significantly reduce their use of steroids, which can be life changing.

The other area with potential to make a big impact is in early lung disease, before significant lung damage has occurred. We currently have no therapies to target patients early in the course of COPD to slow the development of emphysema, which occurs over many years. Being able to do this will first require that as health care systems, we improve our ability to identify patients at an earlier stage of disease. It also means that regulatory agencies, such as the Food and Drug Administration, will need to expand the type of end points they are willing to examine for clinical trials. The FDA has traditionally favored lung function as a primary end point for pulmonary studies. However, even in the setting of significant disease, lung function decline may occur quite slowly. This means that clinical trials testing new medications are more likely to need large numbers of patients and potentially many years to conduct. Other types of clinical trial end points, such as data derived from CT scans, could make trials more feasible and make it easier for new medications to be brought to market.

Another way to spur the expansion of new treatments is through new models of drug development. One of the most fascinating case studies of drug development in the twenty-first century centers around new treatments for cystic fibrosis. In 1998, the median age of survival for a patient with CF was 32 years, thanks to advances in treatments, most notably lung transplants. But a bigger breakthrough was needed. At the time, pharmaceutical companies were hesitant to invest in rare diseases due to the low potential for profit. Robert Beall, then the president and CEO of the Cystic Fibrosis Foundation, forged a new model for drug development based on venture philanthropy. Where nonprofits had traditionally focused their research dollars on academic research, Beall took the approach of partnering with a major pharmaceutical company.

Beall convinced Aurora Biosciences (now Vertex Pharmaceuticals) to partner with the foundation to discover compounds that might correct the core genetic defect in people with CF. The proposal was to use what at the time was a fairly new technique, high-throughput screening, to test over 200,000 potential compounds in lab dishes for their ability to activate the CFTR protein, targeting the most common mutation, called *delta F508*. The most promising compound, a drug called ivacaftor (Kalydeco) was moved into clinical trials. In 2012, the FDA approved ivacaftor for treatment of CF patients carrying the delta F508 mutation. While this particular drug treats only a minority of the CF population, now several combination therapies are available that help the majority of patients with CF. In 2014, the foundation sold royalty rights for CF treatments developed with Vertex for $3.3 billion, equipping the foundation with an extraordinary level of funding for a philanthropic organization. This development approach could catalyze treatment advances for patients with other diseases as well.

The Future of Lung Health

The COVID-19 pandemic has highlighted everything we don't know about the lung. While we have guidance from prior research on how to best support lungs that have been injured, I wish we knew even more. Some studies suggest that once a patient becomes mechanically ventilated, the mortality rate from COVID-19 may be as high as 70 percent. We are also beginning to see patients with persistent symptoms and lung impairment after they have cleared the infection. We will most certainly be facing a new form of chronic respiratory disease. Yet with these illnesses comes a new level of awareness about the importance of lung health and the importance of preserving it.

Now is the time to invest in research focused on understanding lung disease and developing treatments, so that we will be better prepared in the future. Threats to lung health were already lurking, even before COVID-19. Air pollution in certain parts of the world are already at dangerous levels. We must take air pollution and protection of air quality more seriously than we ever have before. The number of youth using tobacco products has reached epidemic proportions. We must proactively protect the lungs of our children and adolescents now. As a medical community, we have become complacent. We need to recognize the warning signs of lung injury much earlier. Spirometry is not just a test of lung health, but rather of human health. It is the fifth vital sign. The number of threats to human lung health increases daily. We can do better. We must do better.

Acknowledgments

A host of people deserve my appreciation for their aid in making this book possible. All of my patients through the years have gifted me a firsthand education in diagnosing and treating lung disease that inspired the book. Several of my academic colleagues read chapters and provided important content feedback. These include Thomas Sisson, Kevin Flaherty, and Douglas Arenberg. I owe a huge debt of gratitude to two colleagues in particular, Jeffrey Curtis and Wassim Labaki. They are both excellent writers in their own right, and each painstakingly edited the entire book. The first draft was also read by one of my patients, Maryann Nordhauser, whose enthusiasm for the project provided much needed encouragement.

Conversations with several other colleagues over the years have also helped me to frame many of the concepts I have discussed, particularly around the meaning of lung health and lung disease. These include Robert Dickson, Mark Dransfield,

ACKNOWLEDGMENTS

George Washko, and Ravi Kalhan. My mentor, Fernando J. Martinez, has always provided incredible guidance, without which this book would not have been possible. This list also includes colleagues at the National Institutes of Health and in particular the Lung Division of the National Heart, Lung and Blood Institute (NHLBI), who are passionate about the pursuit of understanding lung disease and improving human health.

I would be remiss not to mention colleagues at the American Lung Association, COPD Foundation, American Thoracic Society, and GOLD organizations who have helped provide me the platform from which to write this book. In particular, the American Lung Association's communications team, Allison MacMunn and Stephanie Goldina, and CEO Harold Wimmer were instrumental in giving me a voice that allowed this book to be written.

I also owe a debt of gratitude to my editor, Matt Weiland, at W. W. Norton for having faith in me as an author, as well as to my agent, Howard Yoon, for his wisdom throughout this process.

Finally, I must thank my father, who gave me the confidence to pursue medicine, and my mother, husband, and son, who gave me the needed time and space to finish this work. They are my daily inspiration to make the world a better place.

Notes

Chapter 1: How the Lungs Work

1. Prange HD. Laplace's law and the alveolus: A misconception of anatomy and a misapplication of physics. *Adv Physiol Educ.* 2003;27:34–40.
2. Suresh GK, Soll RF. Overview of surfactant replacement trials. *J Perinatol.* 2005;25 Suppl 2:S40–4.
3. Prisk GK, Guy HJ, Elliott AR, West JB. Inhomogeneity of pulmonary perfusion during sustained microgravity on SLS-1. *J Appl Physiol.* 1994;76:1730–8.
4. Taylor AT. High-altitude illnesses: Physiology, risk factors, prevention, and treatment. *Rambam Maimonides Med J.* 2011;2:e0022.

Chapter 2: The Battle Within

1. Venkataraman A, Bassis CM, Beck JM, et al. Application of a neutral community model to assess structuring of the human lung microbiome. *mBio.* 2015;6(1):e02284–14.
2. Sigurs N, Gustafsson PM, Bjarnason R, et al. Severe respiratory syncytial virus bronchiolitis in infancy and asthma and allergy at age 13. *Amer J Respir Crit Care Med.* 2005;171:137–41.

NOTES

3. Li W, Wong SK, Li F, et al. Animal origins of the severe acute respiratory syndrome coronavirus: Insight from ACE2-S-protein interactions. *J Virol*. 2006;80:4211–19.

4. Sakurai A, Sasaki T, Kato S, et al. Natural history of asymptomatic SARS-CoV-2 infection. *N Engl J Med*. 2020;383:885–86.

5. Huang Y, Tan C, Wu J, et al. Impact of coronavirus disease 2019 on pulmonary function in early convalescence phase. *Respir Res*. 2020;21:163.

6. Thompson, et al. Interim Estimates of Vaccine Effectiveness of BNT162b2 and mRNA-1273 COVID-19 Vaccines in Preventing SARS-CoV-2 Infection Among Health Care Personnel, First Responders, and Other Essential and Frontline Workers—Eight US Locations, December 2020–March 2021. MMWR 2021;70(13):495–500. https://www.cdc.gov/mmwr/volumes/70/wr/mm7013e3.htm

7. Podolosky SH. *Pneumonia before antibiotics*. Baltimore, MD: The Johns Hopkins University Press; 2006.

8. Global Tuberculosis Report 2020. World Health Organization. Geneva, 2020.

Chapter 3: Protecting Your Lungs for Life

1. Lange P, Celli B, Agusti A, et al. Lung-function trajectories leading to chronic obstructive pulmonary disease. *N Engl J Med*. 2015;373:111–22.

2. Narayanan M, Owers-Bradley J, Beardsmore CS, et al. Alveolarization continues during childhood and adolescence: New evidence from helium-3 magnetic resonance. *Amer J Respir Crit Care Med*. 2012;185:186–91; Narayanan M, Beardsmore CS, Owers-Bradley J, et al. Catch-up alveolarization in ex-preterm children: Evidence from (3)He magnetic resonance. *Amer J Respir Crit Care Medicine*. 2013;187:1104–9.

3. Bui DS, Lodge CJ, Burgess JA, et al. Childhood predictors of lung function trajectories and future COPD risk: A prospective cohort study from the first to the sixth decade of life. *Lancet Respir Med*. 2018;6:535–44.

4. Davidson LM, Berkelhamer SK. Bronchopulmonary dysplasia: Chronic lung disease of infancy and long-term pulmonary outcomes. *J Clin Med*. 2017;6:4.

5. Bronstein JM, Wingate MS, Brisendine AE. Why is the U.S. preterm birth rate so much higher than the rates in Canada, Great Britain, and Western Europe? *Int J Health Serv*. 2018;48:622–40.

6. World Health Organization Global Strategy for Women's, Children's and Adolescents' Health (2016–2030): 2018 Monitoring Report: Current status and strategic priorities; 2018.

7. Postma DS, Bush A, van den Berge M. Risk factors and early origins of chronic obstructive pulmonary disease. *Lancet*. 2015;385:899–909.

8. McEvoy CT, Spindel ER. Pulmonary effects of maternal smoking on the fetus and child: Effects on lung development, respiratory morbidities, and life long lung health. *Paediatr Respir Rev*. 2017;21:27–33.

9. Control CfD. Pregnancy Risk Assessment Monitoring System, PRAMS, Prevalence of Selected Maternal and Child Health Indicators for all PRAMS sites, 2012–2015;2015.

10. Cunningham J, Dockery DW, Speizer FE. Maternal smoking during pregnancy as a predictor of lung function in children. *Am J Epidemiol*. 1994;139:1139–52.

11. Wongtrakool C, Wang N, Hyde DM, Roman J, Spindel ER. Prenatal nicotine exposure alters lung function and airway geometry through alpha7 nicotinic receptors. *Am J Respir Cell Mol Biol*. 2012;46:695–702.

12. Farsalinos KE, Spyrou A, Stefopoulos C, et al. Nicotine absorption from electronic cigarette use: comparison between experienced consumers (vapers) and naïve users (smokers). *Scientific Reports* 2015;5:11269.

13. McEvoy CT, Schilling D, Clay N, et al. Vitamin C supplementation for pregnant smoking women and pulmonary function in their newborn infants: A randomized clinical trial. *JAMA*. 2014;311:2074–82.

14. McEvoy CT, Shorey-Kendrick LE, Milner K, et al. Oral vitamin C (500 mg/d) to pregnant smokers improves infant airway function at 3 months (VCSIP): A randomized trial. *Amer J Respir Crit Care Med*. 2019;199:1139–47.

15. Abramovici A, Gandley RE, Clifton RG, et al. Prenatal vitamin C and E supplementation in smokers is associated with reduced placental abruption and preterm birth: A secondary analysis. *BJOG*. 2015;122:1740–7.

16. Rumbold A, Ota E, Nagata C, Shahrook S, Crowther CA. Vitamin C supplementation in pregnancy. *Cochrane Database Syst Rev*. 2015:CD004072.

17. Amati F, Hassounah S, Swaka A. The impact of Mediterranean dietary patterns during pregnancy on maternal and offspring health. *Nutrients*. 2019;11(5):1098; Bedard A, Northstone K, Henderson AJ, Shaheen SO. Mediterranean diet during pregnancy and childhood respiratory and atopic outcomes: Birth cohort study. *Eur Respir J*. 2020;55(3):1901215.

18. Stinson LF, Payne MS, Keelan JA. A critical review of the bacterial baptism hypothesis and the impact of cesarean delivery on the infant microbiome. *Front Med (Lausanne)*. 2018;5:135.

19. Cushing AH, Samet JM, Lambert WE, et al. Breastfeeding reduces risk of respiratory illness in infants. *Am J Epidemiol*. 1998;147:863–70.

20. Güngör D, Nadaud P, LaPergola CC, et al. Infant milk-feeding practices and food allergies, allergic rhinitis, atopic dermatitis, and asthma throughout the life span: A systematic review. *Am J Clin Nutr*. 2019;109:772S–99S.

21. World Health Organization. Pneumonia the Forgotten Killer of Children. 2006; Savran O, Ulrik CS. Early life insults as determinants of chronic obstructive pulmonary disease in adult life. *Int J Chron Obstruct Pulmon Dis*. 2018;13:683–93.

22. Korppi M, Piippo-Savolainen E, Korhonen K, Remes S. Respiratory morbidity 20 years after RSV infection in infancy. *Ped Pulm*. 2004;38:155–60.

23. Jackson DJ, Gangnon RE, Evans MD, et al. Wheezing rhinovirus illnesses in early life predict asthma development in high-risk children. *Amer J Respir Crit Care Med*. 2008;178:667–72.

24. Grant T, Brigham EP, McCormack MC. Childhood origins of adult lung disease as opportunities for prevention. *J Allergy Clin Immunol Pract*. 2020;8:849–58.

25. Eisner MD, Anthonisen N, Coultas D, et al. An official American Thoracic Society public policy statement: Novel risk factors and the global burden of chronic obstructive pulmonary disease. *Amer J Respi Crit Care Med*. 2010;182:693–718.

26. Burbank AJ, Peden DB. Assessing the impact of air pollution on childhood asthma morbidity: How, when, and what to do. *Curr Opin Allergy Clin Immunol*. 2018;18:124–31.

27. Cullen KA, Gentzke AS, Sawdey MD, et al. e-Cigarette Use among Youth in the United States, 2019. *JAMA*. 2019;322:2095–103.

28. Kong G, Morean ME, Cavallo DA, Camenga DR, Krishnan-Sarin S. Reasons for electronic cigarette experimentation and discontinuation among adolescents and young adults. *Nicotine Tob Res*. 2015;17:847–54.

29. Goriounova NA, Mansvelder HD. Short- and long-term consequences of nicotine exposure during adolescence for prefrontal cortex neuronal network function. *Cold Spring Harb Perspect Med*. 2012;2(12):a012120.

30. Hamberger ES, Halpern-Felsher B. Vaping in adolescents: Epidemiology and respiratory harm. *Curr Opin Pediatr.* 2020;32:378–83.

31. Bein K, Leikauf GD. Acrolein—a pulmonary hazard. *Mol Nutr Food Res.* 2011;55:1342–60.

32. Bhatta DN, Glantz SA. Association of e-cigarette use with respiratory disease among adults: A longitudinal analysis. *Am J Prev Med.* 2020;58:182–90.

33. Gray, et al. High-dose and low-dose varenicline for smoking cessation in adolescents: a randomized, placebo-controlled trial. *Lancet Child Adolesc Health.* 2020; 4(11):837–845. See also http://labeling.pfizer.com/ShowLabeling.aspx?id=557.

34. Homa DM, Neff LJ, King BA, et al. Vital signs: Disparities in nonsmokers' exposure to secondhand smoke—United States, 1999–2012. *MMWR.* 2015;64:103–8.

35. Bui DS, Lodge CJ, Burgess JA, et al. Childhood predictors of lung function trajectories and future COPD risk: A prospective cohort study from the first to the sixth decade of life. *Lancet Respir Med.* 2018;6:535–44.

36. Tashkin DP. Marijuana and lung disease. *Chest.* 2018;154:653–63.

37. Blanc PD. Occupation and COPD: A brief review. *J Asthma.* 2012;49:2–4.

38. Sadhra S, Kurmi OP, Sadhra SS, Lam KB, Ayres JG. Occupational COPD and job exposure matrices: A systematic review and meta-analysis. *Int J Chron Obstruct Pulmon Dis.* 2017;12:725–34.

39. Su CP, Syamlal G, Tamers S, Li J, Luckhaupt SE. Workplace secondhand tobacco smoke exposure among U.S. nonsmoking workers, 2015. *MMWR.* 2019;68:604–7.

40. Pirela S, Molina R, Watson C, et al. Effects of copy center particles on the lungs: A toxicological characterization using a Balb/c mouse model. *Inhal Toxicol.* 2013;25:498–508; Gallardo M, Romero P, Sanchez-Quevedo MC, Lopez-Caballero JJ. Siderosilicosis due to photocopier toner dust. *Lancet.* 1994;344:412–3; Armbruster C, Dekan G, Hovorka A. Granulomatous pneumonitis and mediastinal lymphadenopathy due to photocopier toner dust. *Lancet.* 1996;348:690; Nakadate T, Yamano Y, Adachi C, et al. A cross sectional study of the respiratory health of workers handling printing toner dust. *Occup Environ Med.* 2006;63:244–9.

41. Reponen T, Lockey J, Bernstein DI, et al. Infant origins of childhood asthma associated with specific molds. *J Allergy Clin Immunol.*

2012;130:639–44.e5.

42. Benck LR, Cuttica MJ, Colangelo LA, et al. Association between cardiorespiratory fitness and lung health from young adulthood to middle age. *Amer J Respir Crit Care Med.* 2017;195:1236–43.

43. Kalhan R, Tran BT, Colangelo LA, et al. Systemic inflammation in young adults is associated with abnormal lung function in middle age. *PLoS One.* 2010;5:e11431; Church TS, Barlow CE, Earnest CP, Kampert JB, Priest EL, Blair SN. Associations between cardiorespiratory fitness and C-reactive protein in men. *Arterioscler Thromb Vasc Biol.* 2002;22:1869–76; LaMonte MJ, Durstine JL, Yanowitz FG, et al. Cardiorespiratory fitness and C-reactive protein among a tri-ethnic sample of women. *Circulation.* 2002;106:403–6.

44. Sluyter JD, Camargo CA, Waayer D, et al. Effect of monthly, high-dose, long-term vitamin D on lung function: A randomized controlled trial. *Nutrients.* 2017;9(12):1353.

Chapter 4: How Pulmonologists Think

1. Savran O, Ulrik CS. Early life insults as determinants of chronic obstructive pulmonary disease in adult life. *Int J Chron Obstruct Pulmon Dis.* 2018;13:683–93.

2. Fuseini H, Newcomb DC. Mechanisms driving gender differences in asthma. *Curr Allergy Asthma Rep.* 2017;17:19.

3. Puri B, Shankar Raman V. Physical examination: The dying art. *Med J Armed Forces India.* 2017;73:110–1.

4. Roguin A. Rene Theophile Hyacinthe Laënnec (1781–1826): The man behind the stethoscope. *Clin Med Res.* 2006;4:230–5.

5. Gibson G. Spirometry: Then and now. *Breathe.* 2005;1:206–2016.

Chapter 5: A Short Guide to Chronic Lung Diseases

1. Rogalsky DK, Mendola P, Metts TA, Martin WJ, 2nd. Estimating the number of low-income Americans exposed to household air pollution from burning solid fuels. *Environ Health Perspect.* 2014;122:806–10.

2. Han MK, Kim MG, Mardon R, et al. Spirometry utilization for COPD: How do we measure up? *Chest.* 2007;132:403–9.

3. A Randomized Trial of Long-Term Oxygen for COPD with Moderate Desaturation. *N Engl J Med.* 2016;375:1617–27.

4. Wakelee HA, Chang ET, Gomez SL, et al. Lung cancer incidence in never smokers. *J Clin Oncol*. 2007;25:472–8.
5. Thun MJ, Carter BD, Feskanich D, et al. 50-year trends in smoking-related mortality in the United States. *N Engl J Med* .2013;368:351–64.

Chapter 6: The Fifth Vital Sign

1. Petty TL. John Hutchinson's mysterious machine revisited. *Chest*. 2002;121:219S-23S.
2. Petty TL. John Hutchinson's mysterious machine revisited. *Chest*. 2002;121:219S-23S.
3. Mahmood SS, Levy D, Vasan RS, Wang TJ. The Framingham Heart Study and the epidemiology of cardiovascular disease: A historical perspective. *Lancet*. 2014;383:999–1008.
4. World Health Organization. Number of grants for biomedical research by funder, type of grant, duration and recipients. World RePORT. 2019.
5. Gillum LA, Gouveia C, Dorsey ER, et al. NIH disease funding levels and burden of disease. *PLoS One*. 2011;6:e16837.
6. Best RK. Disease politics and medical research funding: Three ways advocacy shapes policy. *Amer Sociol Rev*. 2012;77(5):780–803.
7. Hamanaka RB, Mutlu GM. Particulate matter air pollution: Effects on the cardiovascular system. *Front in Endocrinol*. 2018;9:680.

Illustration Credits

39 Adapted from Liu YC, Kuo RL, Shih SR. COVID-19: The first documented coronavirus pandemic in history. *Biomed J.* 2020;43:328–33.

40 *New England Journal of Medicine*, Camille Ehre, "SARS-CoV-2 Infection of Airway Cells," Volume 383, Issue 1, Page 969. Copyright © 2020 Massachusetts Medical Society. Reprinted with permission from Massachusetts Medical Society.

99 Adapted from Gillum LA, Gouveia C, Dorsey ER, et al. NIH disease funding levels and burden of disease. *PLoS One.* 2011;6:e16837.

Index

Page numbers in italics refer to illustrations.